Praises for The Bragg Back Fitness Program and The Bragg Healthy Lifestyle

These are just a few of the thousands of testimonials we receive yearly, praising The Bragg Health Books for the rejuvenation benefits they reap – physically, mentally and spiritually. We look forward to hearing from you also.

Bragg Healthy Lifestyle, Super Power Breathing and Back Books help make the weak strong and athletes champions.
– Bob Anderson, famous stretching coach • *www.stretching.com*

When I was a young Stanford University gymnastics coach Paul Bragg's words and example inspired me to live a healthy lifestyle. I was twenty-three then; now I'm over sixty-two, and my own health and fitness serves as a living testimonial to Bragg's wisdom, carried on by Patricia, his dedicated Health Crusading daughter.
– Dan Millman, author, *Way of the Peaceful Warrior*
• *www.peacefulwarrior.com*

Paul Bragg saved my life when I attended the Bragg Health Crusade in Oakland. At 15 I was so weak and sickly, that I had to wear a back brace to sit up. I thank The Bragg Healthy Lifestyle for my long, healthy, active life and I love spreading health and fitness.
– Jack LaLanne, Bragg follower & fitness pioneer to 96½
• *www.JackLaLanne.com*

As a youth I had a learning disability and was told I would never read, write or communicate normally. At 14 I dropped out of school and at 17 ended up in Hawaii surfing. My road to recovery led me to Paul Bragg who changed my life by giving me one simple affirmation to repeat: *"I am a genius and I apply my wisdom."* Paul Bragg inspired me to go back to school and get my education and from there miracles happened. I have authored 72 training programs and 40 books and love to crusade around the world thanks to Paul Bragg.
– Dr. John Demartini, Dynamic Health Crusader,
Star in *The Secret* • www

Good health and good sense are two of life's greatest blessings.
– Publilius Syrus, Latin Writer, 42 B.C.

Ⓐ

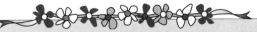

Praises for The Bragg Healthy Lifestyle

The Bragg Healthy Lifestyle teaches you to take control of
your health and build a healthy, fulfilled, long life.
– Mark Victor Hansen, co-creator, *Chicken Soup for the Soul* series

---

Thanks to Bragg Health Books, they were our introduction to
healthy living. We are very grateful to you and your father.
– Marilyn Diamond, co-author, *Fit For Life* – best-seller 40 weeks

---

Bragg Books were my conversion to the healthy way.
– James F. Balch, M.D., co-author,
Prescription for Nutritional Healing

The *Bragg Healthy Lifestyle, Apple Cider Vinegar* and *Miracle
of Fasting* books have changed my life! I lost weight and my
energy levels went through the roof. I look forward to my
fasting days. I think better and am a better husband and father.
Thank you Patricia, this has been a great blessing in my life.
Also, we enjoyed your health sharing at our "AOL" Conference.
– Byron H. Elton, former VP Entertainment, Time Warner AOL

I met Paul Bragg in 1964 at "L" Street Beach in Boston. Both
Paul and his daughter Patricia are dynamic, energetic and
life-changers! They have always been health inspirations to
millions around the world, but especially to me! I gave my first
lecture with them in April 1964, I was 22, I am over 64 now.
Patricia has more energy than any 3 people I know put together
and loves traveling the world for Bragg Health Crusades.
– Dr. David Carmos and Dr. Shawn Miller,
co-authors of *You're Never Too Old To Become Young*

Thank you Patricia for our first meeting in London in 1968.
You gave me your Fasting Book, it got me exercising, brisk
walking and eating more wisely. You were a blessing
God-sent. – Rev. Billy Graham

Our prayers should be for a sound mind in a healthy body.
– Juvenal, Roman Poet active in the early 2nd Century A.D.

B

A laugh is just like sunshine. It freshens all the day. – Heart Warmers

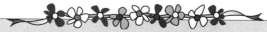

Praises for The Bragg Healthy Lifestyle

I have read your book *Apple Cider Vinegar*. My lower back aches and hip pain are totally gone from 25 years of jogging and martial arts. Like your book says, *"try it and you be the judge."* Well I've tried it and I will always love it. Thank you.
– Kelly Numrich, Saskatchewan, Canada

I have had back issues for the last 30 years. A visit with Patricia brought me more than I expected. It was part of my healing. With the combination of structural integration and Bragg Back Fitness Program, I have found my solution. So much tension is held in our backs that has an impact on everything we do. As a part of my program I am integrating what works and you can too! Our physical form is our projection into the world and our posture allows us to present ourselves in a bright light. Be that bright light!
– Dr. Nick Begich, author/speaker • *www.EarthPulse.com*

Thanks to Paul Bragg and Bragg Health Books, my early years of asthma were cured in one month with the Bragg Healthy Lifestyle living!
– Paul Wenner, Gardenburger creator • *www.Gardenburger.com*

I had the opportunity to sit next to Patricia on a flight from Dallas to Los Angeles. Her honesty about my weight and health really inspired me to make a life change. One year later, I am 85 lbs. lighter and heart rate cut almost in half. Patricia you helped save my life! – Mike Ableman, Texas

Thanks to the Bragg Fasting Book and the Healthy Lifestyle, we are healthy, fit and singing better and staying younger than ever! – The Beach Boys • *www.TheBeachBoys.com*

I have known Patricia Bragg for over 15 years and have always been inspired by her books, her knowledge, and her lifestyle. This book will tell you everything you ever wanted to know about foot health and how your feet affect your overall well-being.
– Richard Diehl, Ph.D., M.Ed., L.Ac., Hawaii

Love begins by taking care of the loved ones at home. – Mother Teresa

Praises for The Bragg Healthy Lifestyle

I give thanks to Paul C. Bragg and his daughter Patricia for their long years of devoted service spreading health and fitness worldwide. It has made a difference in my life and millions of others.– Pat Robertson, Host "700 Club"

How I beat obesity, diabetes, strep and three herniated disks and excruciating pain? The answer was changing to Bragg's Healthy Lifestyle Program! It changed and saved my life! I recovered and also lost over 70 lbs. I received a new life and that is just the beginning because my manhood returned that was lost to diabetes – now that's exciting! On my trip to Honolulu, Hawaii I visited the famous free Bragg Exercise Class at Waikiki Beach. I became so regenerated and happy with new energy that I want the world to join The Bragg Health Crusade. I am deeply thankful to Health Crusaders, Paul and Patricia for my well-being. – Len, Hawaii

I've experienced a beautiful, remarkable, spiritual and physical awakening since reading Bragg Books. I'll never be the same again. – Sandy Tuttle, Ohio

We get letters daily at our Santa Barbara headquarters. We would love to receive a testimonial from you on any blessings, healings and changes you have experienced after following The Bragg Healthy Lifestyle and this book. It's all within your grasp to be in top health. By following this book, you can reap more Super Health and a happy, long fulfilled vital life! It's never too late to begin! Studies show amazing results that were obtained with people in their 80's and 90's. Receive miracles with natural nutrition, exercise and some fasting! Start now!

Daily our prayers & love go out to you, your heart, mind & soul.
With love,

Patricia Bragg

3 John 2

Miracles can happen daily through guidance and prayer! – Patricia Bragg

Bragg
BACK &
FOOT
Fitness Program
Keys to a Pain Free Back & Strong Healthy Feet

PAUL C. BRAGG, N.D., Ph.D.
LIFE EXTENSION SPECIALIST

and

PATRICIA BRAGG
HEALTH CRUSADER & LIFESTYLE EDUCATOR

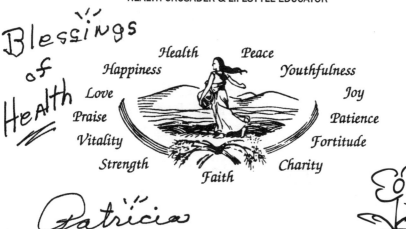

Blessings of Health

Health Peace
Happiness Youthfulness
Love Joy
Praise Patience
Vitality Fortitude
Strength Charity
Faith

Patricia

BECOME
A Health Crusader – for a 100% Healthy World for All!

www.PatriciaBraggBooks.com

Bragg
BACK &
FOOT
Fitness Program
Keys to a Pain Free Back & Strong Healthy Feet

PAUL C. BRAGG, N.D., Ph.D.
LIFE EXTENSION SPECIALIST
and
PATRICIA BRAGG
HEALTH CRUSADER & LIFESTYLE EDUCATOR

Visit our website:
www.PatriciaBraggBooks.com

First Edition MMXXII
ISBN: 978-0-87790-092-4

Library of Congress Cataloging-in-Publication Data on file with publisher

Published in the United States
HEALTH SCIENCE
7127 Hollister Avenue, Suite 25A, Box 249, Santa Barbara, CA 93117
Toll-Free: (833) 408-1122

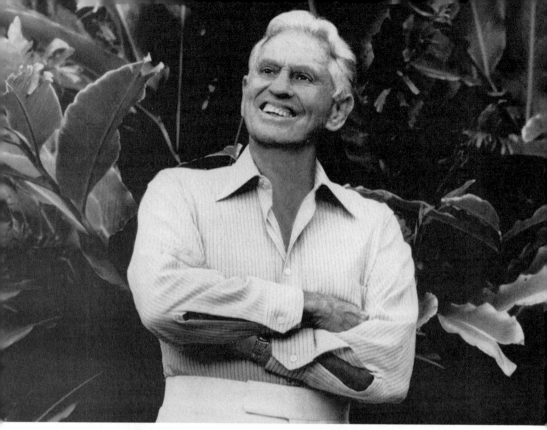

PAUL C. BRAGG, N.D., Ph.D.
World's Leading Healthy Lifestyle Authority

Paul C. Bragg's daughter Patricia and their wonderful, healthy members of the Bragg *Longer Life, Health and Happiness Club* exercised daily on the beautiful Fort DeRussy lawn, at famous Waikiki Beach in Honolulu, Hawaii. On Saturday there were often health lectures on how to live a long, healthy life! The group averaged 50 to 75 per day, depending on the season. From December to March it can go up to 125. Its dedicated leaders carried on the class for over 43 years. Thousands visited the club from around the world and carried the Bragg Health and Fitness Crusade to friends and relatives back home.

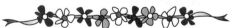

Your body is a non-stop living system, in constant motion 24 hours daily, cleaning, repairing, healing and growing. – Patricia Bragg

To maintain good health, normal weight and increase the good life of radiant health, joy and happiness, the body must be exercised properly (stretching, walking, jogging, biking, swimming, deep breathing, good posture) and nourished with healthy foods. – Paul C. Bragg, N.D., Ph.D.

iii

❀ Cautionary Note and Disclaimer ❀

The information provided here is for educational purposes only. Any decision on your part to read, listen and use this information is your personal choice. The information in this book is not meant to be used to diagnose, prescribe or treat any illness. Please discuss any changes you wish to make to your medical treatment with a qualified, licensed health care provider.

If you are taking medication to control your blood sugar or blood pressure, you may need to reduce the dosage if you significantly restrict your carbohydrate intake. This is best done under the care and supervision of an experienced and qualified licensed health care provider. Anyone who has any other serious illness such as cardiovascular disease, cancer, kidney or liver disease needs to exercise caution if making dietary changes. You should consult your physician for guidance. If you are pregnant or lactating, you should not overly restrict protein or fat intake. Also, young children and teens have much more demanding nutrient needs and should NOT have their protein or fat intake overly restricted.

The information presented in this book is in no way intended as medical advice or a substitute for medical counseling. It is intended only to provide the opinions and ideas of the authors. It is sold with the understanding that the authors are not engaged in rendering medical, health or any other kind of professional services in this book. The reader should consult his or her medical doctor, or any other competent professional, before adopting any of the suggestions in this book, or drawing inferences from it.

The authors disclaim any responsibility for any liability, loss or risk, personal or otherwise, which is incurred as a consequence, directly or indirectly, of the use and application of the contents of this book.

Please consult your physician before beginning this program, and use all of the information the authors suggest in conjunction with the guidance and care of your physician. Your physician should be aware of all medical conditions that you may have, as well as medications and supplements you are taking.

BRAGG
BACK & FOOT
Fitness Program

To preserve health is a moral and religious duty, for health is the basis for all social virtues. We can no longer be as useful when not well.
– Dr. Samuel Johnson, Father of Dictionaries, 1709-1784

Contents

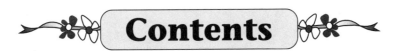

Contents

Contents

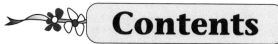

Make your two feet your best friends as they carry you.
– J. M. Barrie, author of "Peter Pan"

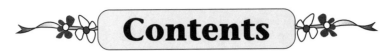

Contents

Contents

Contents

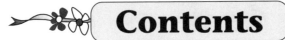

*Bragg Health Books are silent health teachers and your friends –
never tiring, ready night or day to help you help yourself to health!*

Chapter 1

Your Miracle Body Mechanics
Bones, joints, muscles & skeletal system

If you suddenly removed the poles from a circus tent, the tent would collapse. The typical adult skeleton is comprised of 206 bones that support the softer parts of the body and give the body its general shape. If the spine, corresponding to the main pole of the tent, and the other supporting bones (or *poles*) were suddenly removed, the body would sink to the ground in a shapeless mass.

The spinal column, the master bones of the human body, is composed of 26 hollow cylinders of bone called *vertebrae*. If you string 26 spools of thread on a stiff wire in the shape of a very open letter "S," you've constructed something resembling the miracle human spinal column.

The skull, which is supported by the spinal column, is made up of 29 flat bones. The round part of the skull that encases the brain is called the cranium, which consists of eight bones. The face, including the lower jaw, consists of 14 bones. There are three tiny bones in each ear. There is a single bone, the hyoid, in the throat.

The chest is composed of 25 bones: a single breastbone, called the sternum, and 24 ribs. All ribs are attached to the spinal column. The upper seven pairs of ribs (14 bones) are attached to the spinal column at the back and the sternum in front. The next three pairs (six bones) attach only to the spinal column, curve around the front of the thorax (chest) but do not meet the sternum. The two lowest pairs of ribs (four bones), called the *floating ribs*, extend from the spine only partway toward the front. There are two collarbones (clavicles), which are attached to the sternum in front and to the two shoulder blades (scapulas) at each side.

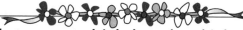

You are what you eat, drink, breathe, think, say and do!
– Patricia Bragg, Pioneer Health Crusader

Keep your bones healthy and youthful with exercise and good nutrition.

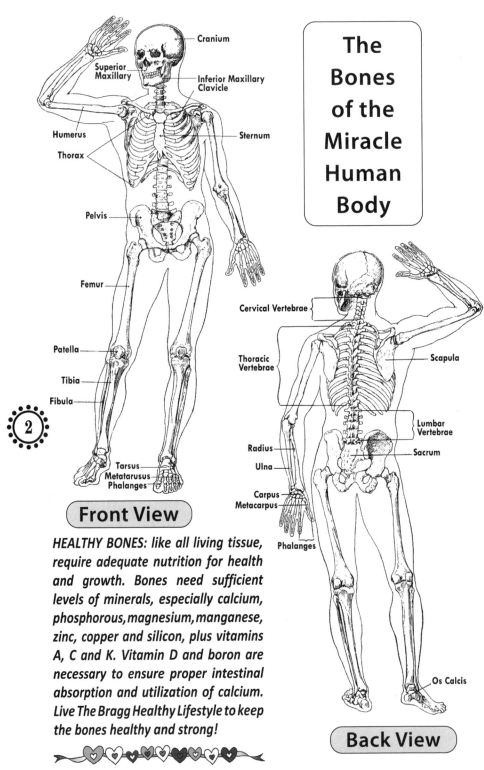

The Bones of the Miracle Human Body

Front View

- Cranium
- Superior Maxillary
- Inferior Maxillary Clavicle
- Humerus
- Thorax
- Sternum
- Pelvis
- Femur
- Patella
- Tibia
- Fibula
- Tarsus
- Metatarusus
- Phalanges

Back View

- Cervical Vertebrae
- Thoracic Vertebrae
- Scapula
- Lumbar Vertebrae
- Radius
- Sacrum
- Ulna
- Carpus
- Metacarpus
- Phalanges
- Os Calcis

HEALTHY BONES: like all living tissue, require adequate nutrition for health and growth. Bones need sufficient levels of minerals, especially calcium, phosphorous, magnesium, manganese, zinc, copper and silicon, plus vitamins A, C and K. Vitamin D and boron are necessary to ensure proper intestinal absorption and utilization of calcium. Live The Bragg Healthy Lifestyle to keep the bones healthy and strong!

Every man is the builder of a temple, called his body. We are all our own sculptors and painters, and our material is our own flesh, blood and bones.
– Henry David Thoreau, American Philosopher, "Walden Pond," 1854

2

Your Body's Strong, Hard-Working Bones

Each arm consists of one upper arm bone, the humerus, and two forearm bones, the ulna and the radius. There are eight bones in each wrist, the carpi, each with a different anatomical name and function. Five bones, called metacarpi, connect the wrist with the fingers, which are composed of 14 bones, called the phalanges (two in the thumb, three in each finger).

Connected to the lowest part of the spinal column (the sacrum and coccyx) are the two hip bones (coxa), the broadest bones of the skeleton. Each connects with a thigh bone (femur), the thigh bones being the longest, strongest and heaviest bones of the body. In each leg, the kneecap (patella) covers the joint attaching the thigh bone to the two lower leg bones, the shinbone (tibia) and its smaller companion, the fibula.

There are seven bones, the tarsi, in each ankle (larger than those in the wrist). Five bones, called metatarsi, form the foot arch, connecting the ankle and toes. As in the fingers, there are 14 bones (called phalanges) in the toes of each foot, two in the big toe and three ③ in each of the other toes. **Your body is a miracle of working bones!**

Major Foot Bones

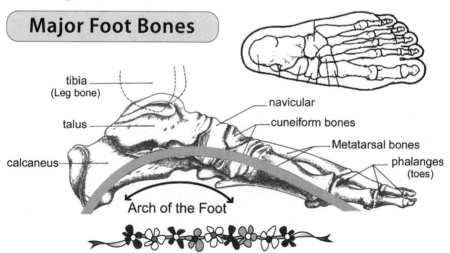

tibia (Leg bone)

talus

calcaneus

navicular

cuneiform bones

Metatarsal bones

phalanges (toes)

Arch of the Foot

Each foot has 26 movable bones, 25% of the body's bones.

Treatment of the feet to improve comfort and function will favorably affect other parts of the body. – Elizabeth H. Roberts, D.P.M.

Health success depends on your strong backbone, not your wishbone.

Composition of the Bones

To be healthy and strong, both cartilage and bones need a full daily ration of organic calcium, phosphorus, magnesium and manganese (natural sources of these minerals will be given in a later section on nutrition).

The long bones, such as the arms and legs, are generally cylindrical in shape, and the long portion is called the shaft. The ends of these bones are thicker and are shaped to fit into the ends of the adjoining bones to form the various types of joints described in the preceding section. The short bones, such as those of the wrist and ankle, are composed mostly of a thick shaft of elastic, spongy material inside a thin covering of hard bone material. Flat bones, such as the ribs, are made up of spongy material between plates of hard bone.

Bones – What's Inside and Outside

A cross section of the bone shows 2 main types of material which it is composed of. The *hard outer layer* that gives bone its shape and strength consists primarily of chemical compounds of calcium and phosphorus. Bones and teeth contain 99% of the body's calcium. This is why calcium is required more than any other mineral for body tissue repair.

The *soft inner part* of the bone is called marrow. Most bone marrow is yellowish in color, made up of fat cells and serving as a storage depot for fat which can be converted into energy as the body's needs require. Toward the ends of the long bones and generally throughout the interior of the flat bones (such as the skull and the spinal column), patches and streaks of reddish tissue show in the marrow. These are the vital manufacturing centers of red blood cells (or corpuscles), which transport life-giving oxygen throughout the body! The white blood corpuscles, which combat infection, are also produced in the bone marrow.

Bone is made mostly of collagen, but also contains calcium phosphate and calcium carbonate, minerals that add strength and harden the framework. The combination of calcium and collagen gives the bone its strength and flexibility. – www.eMedicineHealth.com

Bones Help Protect Your Vital Organs

Bones also protect the softer parts of the body, especially the vital organs. The skull forms a strong case for the soft gray matter of the brain. Two bony sockets in front of the skull protect the eyes. The spinal column is a bony tube that safeguards the delicate, vital spinal cord.

The ribs form a hard, elastic framework that protects the heart and lungs. If a person had no ribs and bumped into something, even a small bump might collapse the lungs or damage the heart. The lower rib cage shelters the back and sides, kidneys and major organs of the upper digestive system. The important protecting ribs are supported by the spinal column. The pelvic bones, which include the base of the spinal column (sacrum and coccyx) and the hip bones, protect the bladder and the vital reproductive organs.

Bone Structure of the Spinal Column

How is this marvelous pivot of the human skeleton constructed? To illustrate some of its functions, we have likened it to the ridgepole of a house or the main pole of a tent. The spine is not a single rigid bone; if it was, the motions of the human body would be very limited. The spine is a flexible column composed of 26 bones – 24 small vertebrae from the base of the skull to the pelvic region, the sacrum (which is actually the natural fusion of five embryonic vertebrae into a wedge-shaped bone that forms the back of the pelvis) and the coccyx (or tail bone, the small triangular bone of four fused embryonic vertebrae at the base of the sacrum).

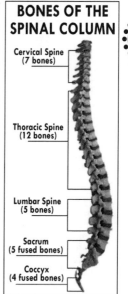

BONES OF THE SPINAL COLUMN

5

Cervical Spine
(7 bones)

Thoracic Spine
(12 bones)

Lumbar Spine
(5 bones)

Sacrum
(5 fused bones)

Coccyx
(4 fused bones)

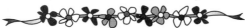

Viewed from the side, an adult spine has a natural S-shaped curve. The neck (cervical) and low back (lumbar) regions have a slight concave curve, and thoracic and sacral regions have a gentle convex curve. The curves work like a coiled spring to absorb shock, maintain balance and allow range of motion throughout the spinal column. – MayfieldClinic.com

The Body's Miracle-Working Joints

Except for the U-shaped hyoid bone of the throat, every bone in the body miraculously is connected, or articulates, with another. The spinal column is the main miracle working pivot of the entire body skeletal system.

The point at which two bones meet, is known as a joint. The joints of the cranium, the part of the skull that houses the brain, are immovable. Those that join the ribs and spine are partially movable. Movement is even more limited in the sacroiliac joints, connecting the base of the spine with the hip bones, where the whole weight of the trunk is supported. Sacroiliac pain (#1 back problem) occurs when the tough, resistant ligaments that hold these joints together weaken under continued or unusual stress, such as lifting a heavy object, a sudden body twist, or the strain from trying to raise a jammed window, etc. (Spine Motion Exercises will help strengthen these important ligaments.)

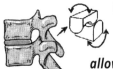

The Six Major Joints of the Body

GLIDING JOINTS: movement at this joint consists of two flat surfaces that slide over each other to allow movement.

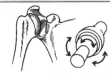

BALL-AND-SOCKET JOINTS: allows movement in 3 planes and is the most mobile of the joints.

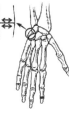

ELLIPSOID JOINTS: allow bending and extending, rocking from side to side, but rotation is limited.

PIVOT JOINTS: permit the bones to rotate like a key turning in a lock. The elbow is a combination of pivot joint and hinge joint.

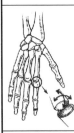

VERTEBRAE & SADDLE JOINTS: allows moving forward, backward and sideways.

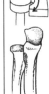

HINGE JOINTS: Permits backward and forward movement like door hinges.

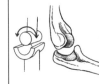

Movable Body Joints – Your Strong Servants

There are six main types of movable joints in the body and, as you will recognize from their names, these human joints have served as patterns that humans have adapted mechanically. **Ball-and-socket joints,** connecting the shoulder to the arm and the hip to the leg, permit the widest range of movement. **Hinge joints,** like those of the knees, fingers and toes, allow bending back and forth only. A **pivot joint** permits the bones to rotate at the joint like a key turning in a lock, such as at the wrists and ankles and the joints at the base of fingers and toes.

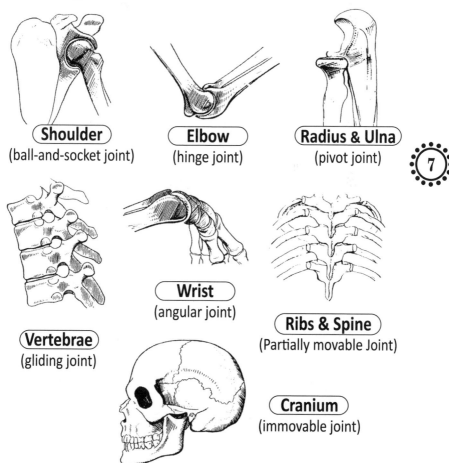

Shoulder
(ball-and-socket joint)

Elbow
(hinge joint)

Radius & Ulna
(pivot joint)

Wrist
(angular joint)

Vertebrae
(gliding joint)

Ribs & Spine
(Partially movable Joint)

Cranium
(immovable joint)

These are the types of faithful, hard working miracle joints in your body. Between the movable ones, a clear amber lubricant called synovial fluid keeps the joint moving easily. When inorganic minerals from toxic acid crystals or hard drinking water begin to replace this fluid, the joints become stiff, arthritic and painful, and then the body feels miserable.

The elbow is a combination of a pivot joint and a hinge joint, allowing one bone of the forearm to rotate about the other as well as providing a bending motion. *Saddle joints,* like those of the vertebrae, allow movement in all directions that is of a more limited sort than that of ball-and-socket joints. These saddle joints permit limited movement forward, backward and sideways. Although each vertebra moves only slightly on the one adjoining it, the combined movement of 26 vertebrae bones make the column flexible as a whole.

An *ellipsoid joint* is a joint with two axes of motion through the same bone. Examples of this joint can be found in the wrists and the in the fingers. A *gliding or plane joint* is a common type of synovial joint formed between bones that meet at flat or nearly flat surfaces. Gliding joints allow bones to glide past one another in any direction along the plane of the joint – up and down, left and right, and diagonally. There are many gliding joints between the bones of the wrist; between the bones of the palm; between the bones of the ankle; and between the bones of the foot. These small bones form many flattened facets between one another to provide miracle flexibility to the hands and feet.

Nature lubricates your joints with precious synovial fluid, which is permanently encased in a membrane. The natural supply of this fluid is ample for a lifetime, but proper diet is important to maintain its consistency, by drinking ample purified distilled water and avoiding hard and fluoridated water and other substances containing toxic inorganic minerals, which will be discussed later.

Always remember you have these vitally important reasons for following The Bragg Healthy Lifestyle:

- The ironclad natural health laws of Mother Nature.
- Your common sense, which tells you that you are doing right.
- Your aim to make your health better and your life longer.
- Your resolve to prevent illness so that you may enjoy life each day.
- You will retain your faculties and be hale, hearty, active and useful far beyond the ordinary length of years.
- You will also possess superior mental and physical powers!
- By making healthy living an art, you will be youthful at any age.

Cartilage – Your Joints' Shock Absorbers

Also lining the bone surfaces of the joints is a tough, springy tissue called *cartilage*, which not only prevents the bone surfaces from rubbing against each other, but also acts as an all-important shock absorber. This is particularly important in the spine, where cartilage plates and intervertebral discs (described later) between the vertebrae absorb the shocks of ordinary actions such as walking, sitting and any jars or blows to the spine.

Cartilage is the precursor of bones in the formation of the skeleton in the embryo, and some of it remains as part of the skeletal system. At birth, the *soft* parts of a baby's skull are miracle cartilaginous that allow room for growth of the brain, changing into hard bone like the rest of the skull after the brain has attained full size. Since cartilage is more elastic than rigid bone, some of it remains at the juncture of the ribs and the sternum to allow full flexible lung breathing expansion. Cartilage also remains part of the adult skeleton in semi-rigid tubes that must be kept permanently open, such as the larynx, trachea (windpipe), bronchi, nose and ears.

Cartilage, also called gristle, is often confused with tendons and ligaments. All three are tough white tissues with varying degrees of elasticity and differences in structure and functions. *Cartilage* is embryonic bone without a direct blood supply and is semirigid, still somewhat elastic. *Tendons* are the white, glistening fibrous bands that attach muscles to bones. They have great tensile strength but are not elastic. They contain a few blood vessels and sensory nerves. *Ligaments* are of similar structure but contain elastic fibers that connect two or more bones or cartilages and support certain organs, muscles and fascia (fibrous enveloping tissue).

Tendons and ligaments are part of the muscular system, while cartilage is part of the skeletal system. The three are only classified together when dealing with what scientists are now calling the *musculoskeletal* system.

We must always improve, renew, rejuvenate ourselves; otherwise, we harden. – Johann Wolfgang von Goethe

Toxic Acid Crystals Cement Joints

Toxic acid crystals can cement movable joints in your feet and back and make them stiff and fill them with misery and torment! Stand on any busy street corner and watch the people hobbling along. Their feet, knees, hips, spine and head seem to be cemented, there is no free-swinging movement in their locomotion. Look at their feet and their hunched back. They seem to pick up their feet heavily and lay them down flatly. Their knees seem to be completely cemented and stiff. There is little movement or swinging motion in the hips. Their spines are rigid and so are their heads. All of the elasticity and resiliency seems to have gone out of what should be a smooth, free-swinging body.

Between the movable joints of every bone in the human body, Mother Nature at one time placed an abundant supply of lubrication known as synovial fluid. Take a look at a youngster who is 10 years of age and see the easy movement of every movable joint in the body. What is the reason that at 66 years old we can't have the freedom of motion in our joints that a child of 10 has? There is no reason! Years have nothing to do with the amount of synovial fluid that makes the joints move freely and easily. **There is one main thing that cements your movable joints and that is toxic acid crystals!**

Age is not toxic. Just because you live to be 60, 70, 80 or 90, there should be no diminishing of the supply of synovial fluid from age! Mother Nature does not stiffen and cement the joints of one person and not another; it is caused by the accumulation of toxins and acid crystals.

Deposits of Inorganic Minerals and Toxic Acid Crystals Cause Painful Feet!

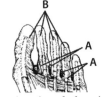

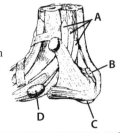

A. Deposited under tendons

B. Under the Achilles tendon

C. Under the heel

D. Under the middle foot

*Inorganic mineral deposits that deposit themselves between the bones of the toes (**A** and **B**).*

Poor Nutrition Causes Toxic Crystal Build-up

Nutrition is as important as exercise for a strong, supple spine and healthy feet. Even Spine Motion Exercises cannot achieve permanent efficiency if you allow vertebral joints to stiffen and calcify with inorganic minerals and toxic acid crystals from improper eating or drinking.

By natural instinct, we eat when hungry, drink when thirsty and breathe air by necessity! Most humans eat way too much food mostly out of habit, not hunger! They have been brainwashed to believe you must have meals by the clock. They don't drink enough water. Thirst mimics their hunger and then they reach for the unhealthy snacks. The average civilized diet is highly acidic in content, upsetting the natural alkaline-acid balance. After each meal, an indigestible, toxic residue remains, which takes the form of toxic acid crystals, inorganic calcium-like mineral substances that cannot be absorbed by the body. So where do these toxic acid crystals go? It is concentrated and crystallized and finds its way into movable body joints. It is a slow unaware process until joints start to give trouble. It takes years of improper eating to bring about heavy concentrations to cause this acid crystal build-up in the movable joints. Gradually, the synovial fluid is displaced by these calcified substances and the joints start becoming stiff and painful. Movable joints are one place where you don't want calcium, especially inorganic calcium, which replaces the vital lubricating synovial fluid with a kind of toxic crystalline cement. When these calcium-like spurs attach themselves on the joints and calcified substances replace the synovial fluid, then pains and aches are felt in the body's movable joints.

This is one of the main reasons why it is important for you to follow the basic rules of natural nutrition that we will outline for you. If you plan your menus along these lines, you will maintain a diet with the proper alkaline-acid balance (which is about $3/5$ alkaline and $2/5$ acid). In general, fruits and vegetables (with a few exceptions) are alkaline forming, while proteins, starches, fats and sugars are acid forming.

How to Flush Out Hardened Acid Crystals

Remember that acid crystals have been building up in your feet and back from the toxic and dead foods you have eaten all of your life, so it has taken a long time. Some people not only build acid crystals but, they also build acid spurs on their foot bones, and these can cause excruciating pain. Sometimes sharp crystals bring on such intense pain because it is no longer possible for the body to break them down. At this point surgery is sometimes the only way to remove spurs that have attached themselves to the movable foot joints. In ordinary cases, toxic acid crystals can be removed by the person themself with a careful hygienic foot plan, as noted in this book. This includes a health hygiene with foot therapy, water treatment, massage, reflexology, exercise, natural nutrition and some fasting.

Fasting is one of the quickest ways to dissolve the acid crystals or spurs from the feet *(fasting also helps normalize weight and blood pressure),* **but** don't expect miracles to happen overnight! These crystals have taken many years to accumulate and sometimes it will take more dedicated months to dissolve them. The first thing to do is to complete a 24-hour fast (water-only) weekly. Then, occasionally take longer fasts. Our book, *The Miracle of Fasting,* covers the hows and whys of fasting in much greater detail than we could go into here. Other Bragg health books that will help you on your quest for perfectly functioning feet are: *Water – The Shocking Truth* and *Apple Cider Vinegar - Miracle Health System.* See back pages for our Bragg booklist.

Also, too much meat in the diet can result in a build-up of acid spurs in the feet! Meat contains a powerful toxin known as uric acid and the heavy meat eater will often suffer from acid crystals. Eggs, cheese and all dairy products are basically on the acidic side, so there must be caution in eating animal products of any kind!

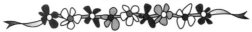

Now learn what and how great benefits a temperate diet will bring along with it. In the first place, you will enjoy good health. – Horace, 65 B.C.

We shall never know all the good that a simple smile can do. – Mother Teresa

Joints Deteriorate without Proper Care

Many things can go wrong when your joints – and especially the cartilage that cushions them – aren't kept healthy. Besides being more susceptible to injury, neglected joints are prone to chronic conditions such as the many different kinds of arthritis (which means inflammation of the joints). An estimated 58.5 million Americans have been told by their physician that they have some form of arthritis, rheumatoid arthritis, gout, lupus or fibromyalgia. Many suffer with stiffness, pain, swelling, instability, deformation, dislocation and reduced mobility in their joints. This damage can result from injury, age, heredity and/or unhealthy living. If you are experiencing severe symptoms, it is important that you consult a health professional to determine the cause and accurately diagnose the discomfort before applying a healing program. In the meantime, there is much that you can do to protect your joints and keep them healthy so that they don't develop problems. And if you do have problems, there are many ways to address them naturally.

13

Natural Ways to Protect and Keep Your Joints Healthy

1. Balanced Diet: The simple principle is that the more excess weight your body has to carry around, the more pressure there is on your joints and the harder they have to work, producing more wear and tear and eventually, pain! It is commonly known that there is a frequent correlation between being overweight and suffering from varied forms of arthritis. A natural, healthy, toxicless diet not only helps you to keep your weight under control, it also maximizes your body's ability to heal itself! Throughout this book we have more details on how to maintain this healthy life-giving diet.

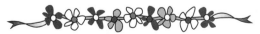

No man can violate Nature's Laws and escape her penalties. – Julian Johnson

 A healthy flexible spine leads to an active, healthy life!

2. Herbs and Supplements – Nature's Healers: You can actually help heal joints naturally, not just control pain. Because a basic symptom of joint trouble is pain caused by inflammation, conventional treatments can include anti-inflammatory drugs such as aspirin, nonsteroidal anti-inflammatory drugs (NSAIDs) like ibuprofen and steroid drugs such as Prednisone. Sometimes a Cortisone injection is prescribed for severe inflammation. While treatments can be helpful in controlling joint pain, it is only a quick and often temporary fix. Aspirin and NSAIDs are hard on the stomach, intestines, kidneys, liver, and actually inhibit the growth of new cartilage!

Your cartilage is miraculously resilient. It changes form when stressed, then springs back to original shape, and with care can be rebuilt and regenerated! Cartilage contains up to 85% water, but the remaining substance includes a wide variety of important sulfur-containing compounds. Sulfur is essential in cartilage and joint repair and it is in many foods (beans, cabbage, garlic, etc.) as well as in supplements. Sulfur is also important and necessary for collagen synthesis and to keep synovial fluid rich and nourishing.

Natural Herbal Remedies for Joint Pain

Herbs and supplements prove helpful in preventing joint disease, reducing pain and restoring injured or inflamed joints. The following herbs and supplements are available at health and vitamin stores and also on-line:

• **DHEA Supplement:** stands for *dehydroepiandrosterone*, a natural substance produced by our adrenal glands. DHEA decreases with age and is linked to age-related joint discomfort, as well as the loss of mobility and sleep.

• **Glucosamine, Chondroitin and MSM:** are essential sulfates to help with joint pain, bone repair, arthritis, and osteoarthritis (see page 92). This combo helps heal and restore cartilage and bones (in caps, liquids, shots).

• **SAM-e:** acts as an analgesic (pain reliever) and has anti-inflammatory properties. It may stimulate cartilage growth and also affects neurotransmitters, such as serotonin, which reduce pain perception. It is best used for osteoarthritis and fibromyalgia.

• **Boswellia Serrata:** has pain-relieving properties. Helps prevent cartilage loss and inhibits autoimmune process.

• **Fish Oil (Omega-3 Fatty Acids):** studies find it significantly decreased joint tenderness and stiffness.

• **Gamma Linolenic Acid (GLA):** is an Omega-6 fatty acid that the body converts into anti-inflammatory chemicals. Trials show significant improvement in joint pain, stiffness and grip strength after 6 months. A study also found that a combination of GLA and Fish Oil significantly reduced the need for pain relievers.

• **Turmeric/Curcumin:** can help reduce joint pain and swelling by blocking the inflammatory enzymes.

• **Capsaicin:** temporarily reduces substance P – a pain transmitter. It can reduce joint pain by 50% after 3 weeks of use. It is available as a topical cream, gel or patch.

• **Zinc, copper, beta-carotene, sulfur, L-lysine, proline and vitamin C:** are important in helping promote and maintain healthy collagen in the body that promotes healthy bones, skin and ligaments. The organic matter in our bones consists mainly of collagen, the "glue" that holds together our skin, tendons, ligaments and bones.

3. Massage and Physiotherapy: can increase vital circulation to help nourish your cartilage, connective tissues and break up unhealthy, painful deposits in joints and tissues. See Alternative Therapies (pages 231-234).

4. Exercise and Movement: Commonly, those who are already experiencing pain are advised to rest, and this feels appropriate because pain usually means *stop!* However, studies show that continued activity in spite of pain actually can lessen pain through release of endorphins and strengthen joints as well. Ice and anti-inflammatory creams, DMSO (pat on), etc., (see page 123) can be used to help lessen discomfort. Hydro (water, hot & cold) therapy also makes easier, pain-free gentle movement possible for many. Regular practice of gentle Yoga, Pilates, Anderson* and Bragg stretching exercises also help maintain healthy flexibility, range of motion and reduce stiffness.

We recommend the book, "Stretching," by Bob Anderson, a top stretching coach and a Bragg Follower. Bob also gives Bragg Super Power Breathing Exercises at Sports Seminars. See web: www.stretching.com

Consider what the Greeks knew and practiced over 5,000 years ago – moderation in all things! The last thing you want to do is overextend yourself and make the problem worse. That's why it is important to keep in close contact with your chiropractor and other health care providers.

According to Dr. John Bland – one of the country's leading arthritis experts at the University of Vermont, *"the most common form of arthritis and osteoarthritis, occurs because of dysfunction of the molecules of connective tissue that line joint surfaces. These collagen molecules can become frayed and irritated by abusive overuse and obesity, basic disuse, or misapplied pressure from an injury or congenitally misaligned joints. A carefully moderated exercise plan, plus diet helps keep weight down and increases muscular strength, flexibility and endurance in order to protect all various body joints from these unhealthy pressures."*

In Some Cases, Prevention May Be Too Late

In advanced cases of joint deterioration, sometimes the only option is surgery. There has been a good deal of success with the following procedures, and research is advancing this practice constantly.

The first kind of surgery is called **osteotomy**, in which damaged bone and tissue are removed and the joint is restored to its proper position. Next are **joint replacement surgeries**, which can be either partial or complete, cemented or uncemented. **Your Board Certified Orthopedist can help to determine which is best for you. We always recommend that you get at least three opinions before committing to any invasive surgery!** The illustrations on the next page show what is involved in total joint replacements.

The advancement of using 3-D technology offers options for making models of a patient's exact bone structure for joint replacement surgeries as well.

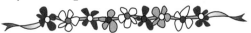

By relieving your body's work of digesting foods, fasting allows your system to rid itself of toxins while facilitating healing! Fasting regularly gives organs a rest and helps reverse the ageing process for a longer and healthier life. Bragg Books were my conversion to the healthy way.
– James Balch, M.D., co-author, "Prescription for Nutritional Healing"

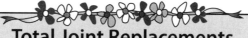

Total Joint Replacements

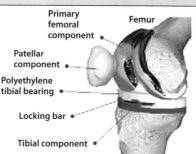

Primary femoral component

Femur

Patellar component

Polyethylene tibial bearing

Locking bar

Tibial component

Total hip surgery removes the damaged femoral head and cartilage from the hip and socket joint, replacing them with prosthesis hip joints made with materials such as metal alloys, plastic and ceramic.

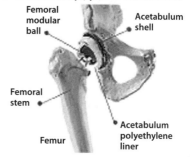

Femoral modular ball

Acetabulum shell

Total knee surgery removes the damaged portions of the femur, tibia, and cartilage, replacing them with a metal and plastic (polyethylene) prosthesis with specially designed weight-bearing surfaces.

Femoral stem

Femur

Acetabulum polyethylene liner

Miracle Spine Ligaments & Muscular System

Although the intervertebral joints add flexibility and sturdiness to the spine, what really holds the spinal column together and in shape are the strong, tough ligaments that weave in and out of the finger-like projections of the spinal arches. Extending from the skull to the sacrum, these powerful, elastic ligaments lace together all the vertebrae and intervertebral discs. Another system of extremely tough ligaments is woven back and forth throughout the sacroiliac area to give the tremendous support necessary to hold together these joints between the hips and spine base (which bear most of the body's weight and that obesity overburdens).

Exercise is vital for those who suffer from stiffness, joint pain, or arthritis. Exercise will help strengthen muscles that support the joints, even when the cartilage is thinning, and helps lubricate joints, allowing them to move more freely. When we are inactive synovial fluid in our joints is the consistency of a thick gel, but once we get moving, liquid becomes more viscous and can do a better job of lubricating our joints and keeping them going smoothly.

Patricia's chance meeting with Jim Bean, seat partner on a flight from LAX to Honolulu saw her going over the "Bragg Back Book." He told her about his successful Birmingham Titanium Hip Resurfacing. From birth defects he suffered pain all his life, after miracle surgery he walked (four hours later) with no pain! – Dr. Colin Poole, Boise, ID
• StLukesOnline.org/health-services/providers/poole-colin

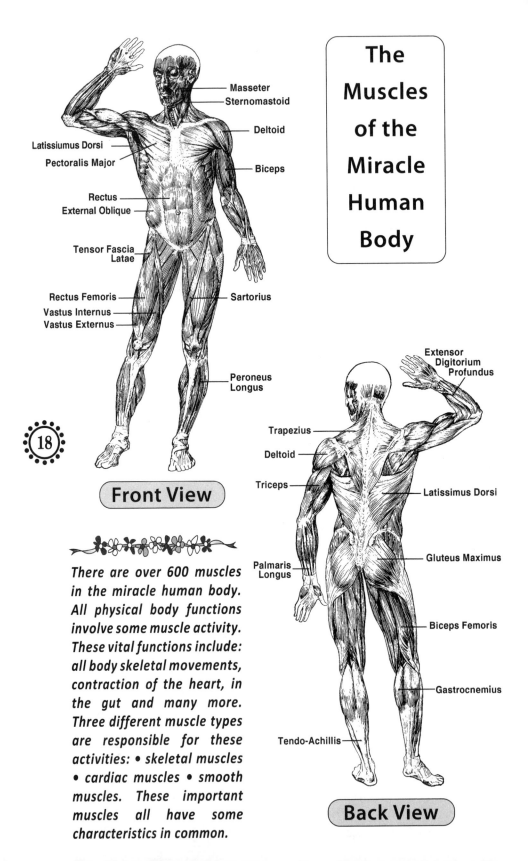

The Muscles of the Miracle Human Body

Front View

- Masseter
- Sternomastoid
- Deltoid
- Latissiumus Dorsi
- Pectoralis Major
- Biceps
- Rectus
- External Oblique
- Tensor Fascia Latae
- Rectus Femoris
- Vastus Internus
- Vastus Externus
- Sartorius
- Peroneus Longus

18

Back View

- Extensor Digitorium Profundus
- Trapezius
- Deltoid
- Triceps
- Latissimus Dorsi
- Palmaris Longus
- Gluteus Maximus
- Biceps Femoris
- Gastrocnemius
- Tendo-Achillis

There are over 600 muscles in the miracle human body. All physical body functions involve some muscle activity. These vital functions include: all body skeletal movements, contraction of the heart, in the gut and many more. Three different muscle types are responsible for these activities: • skeletal muscles • cardiac muscles • smooth muscles. These important muscles all have some characteristics in common.

Muscular System Promotes Health & Flexibility

An elaborate system of muscles is also attached to the vertebrae by tendons to hold the vertebrae in place when the body is at rest, yet allow them to move when the body is in motion. These muscles and the interwoven ligaments around the spinal column are what the Spine Motion Exercises are designed to activate. These exercises are especially designed to achieve and maintain full length and flexibility of the spinal column.

Without muscles to operate the levers, sockets, pivots and gliders of the skeletal system, our skeletons would remain a mere assemblage of static bones. Just as it is the pivot of the skeletal system, the spinal column is the anchor point of the muscular system! Layers of powerful back and abdomen muscles manipulate the body's major movements: bending forward, backward and sideways; reaching upward; lifting; carrying; pulling and pushing. Movements of the head and neck are accomplished by muscles anchored to upper cervical vertebrae. Shoulder and upper-arm muscles anchor to cervical, thoracic and upper lumbar vertebrae, while thigh muscles anchor to the sacrum and coccyx. The muscles operating in our breathing apparatus are anchored to the spine: the diaphragm to lumbar vertebrae and rib muscles to thoracic cervical vertebrae. Pelvic muscles, supporting the viscera and important for good elimination, are anchored to the lower spine.

Even with the operation of all these muscles, the daily activities of the average person does not fully exercise the spine. Its built-in capacity is seldom if ever used, especially in today's under-exercised, malnourished affluent society. We are a civilization of sitters and spectator sportsmen, overfed and malnourished by devitalized, artificial foods.

Please be a good, wise, strict, loving, Mother-like Captain to your Miracle Working Body that is carrying you through life!
– Patricia Bragg, Pioneer Health Crusader

Exercise and Eating Healthy Foods Make Strong Bones and Flexible Muscles

The overall health condition of your spine can determine how fast it will recover from pain and the risk of a condition becoming chronic. Muscles become flabby from lack of regular exercise and tissues depleted from lack of proper nourishment. Unused and misused, the spine then *settles, stiffens and often becomes visibly misshapen.* Dependent on exercise and good circulation in adjacent tissues for their nourishment, cartilage and discs between the vertebrae start deteriorating. The unstretched spinal column *shrinks and ages!* Many people in their 60s and 70s can become three to five inches shorter in height, often called *bent over by old age.*

It is not age, however, that causes the spine to shorten or become bent into abnormal curvature. Deficiency in diet and insufficient or incorrect exercise are so prevalent that many American children and adolescents scuff along with slumped spines, poor posture and no energy. The longer this condition persists, the more pronounced it becomes. That is why it is attributed to age.

If time were the only factor, my Dad's spine would have been fossilized, as a man with great-grandchildren; yet, his spine was just as long, flexible and just as strong in his later years as it was in his youth. Why? Because he knew the vital importance of exercising the spinal column to keep good circulation in his spinal region and of maintaining the muscles and ligaments that hold the spine in place in top tone and fitness. Plus, Dad and I know the essential value of eating natural healthy organic foods that contain the important minerals and vitamins to build strong, healthy bones and cartilage! No spine is any stronger than the food of which it's made, and no spine is any stronger than the exercise it is given, regardless of your calendar years. **Nothing affects your entire life, health, energy and vitality as much as the condition of your spinal column.**

A strong body makes the mind strong. – Thomas Jefferson

Chapter 2

The Importance of Healthy Nutrition

Stop eating unhealthy refined foods

A strong, sturdy, enduring, tireless, painless and ageless feeling back and happy feet are built by a well-nourished, healthy, rich, red bloodstream! Your blood and body are made from the food you eat and the liquids you drink! **Every 90 days you build a complete new bloodstream.** So in 90 days, with careful attention to your food program, you can build a bloodstream that is going to help you cleanse, heal and rebuild a new, strong, back and healthy feet.

To build a strong back, tireless feet and a healthy bloodstream, let's first discuss what *not* to do. The worst enemies of a healthy back, feet and blood are white refined sugars, white refined flours, white rice, alcohol, tobacco, coffee, tea and all soft drinks! (See "Foods to Avoid," page 38.) It's impossible to build a healthy, rich bloodstream, and maintain a healthy back, feet and body out of these unhealthy, toxic materials! **Your health is your greatest wealth! Don't let your body prematurely age and decay! Your body is a miracle instrument, please regard it as such!** You should only put into your body foods that build healthy, strong bones and tendons in all the movable joints of the feet, arms, legs and back!

A good nutritious diet is based on the amount of protective foods that are used in it. For a healthy diet, have ample raw and properly cooked organic vegetables and fresh fruits (page 23). Also have a balance of protein *(vegetarian is best)*, plus minerals, vitamins and enzymes.

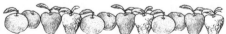

Refined white flour has a long shelf life because it is actually dead; the vital raw wheat germ, one of nature's richest sources of nutrition, having been refined out of it, leaves nothing but empty calories.

Self discipline is your golden key; without it, you can't be happy and healthy. – Maxwell Maltz, M.D. author "Psycho-Cybernetics" and a Bragg Follower

Start Eating Healthy Foods For Super Energy

The *Healthy Plant-Based Daily Food Guide Pyramid* illustration below, represents an ideal way of eating for achieving optimal nutrition, health and longevity! You will notice that this Food Guide Pyramid is based on healthy organic plant-based foods, with emphasis on fruits, vegetables, whole grains, vegetable protein foods, non-dairy calcium foods, raw nuts, seeds and purified water. This is the best diet for building a healthy nervous system, disease prevention and to enjoy longevity. *Eating a diet based on these dietary guidelines will help get the nutrients you need for optimal health!*

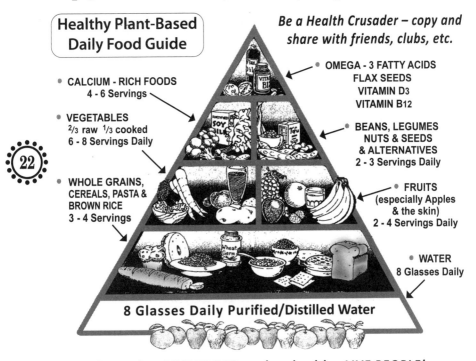

Healthy Plant-Based Daily Food Guide

Be a Health Crusader – copy and share with friends, clubs, etc.

- OMEGA - 3 FATTY ACIDS
  FLAX SEEDS
  VITAMIN D3
  VITAMIN B12

- CALCIUM - RICH FOODS
  4 - 6 Servings

- VEGETABLES
  2/3 raw 1/3 cooked
  6 - 8 Servings Daily

- BEANS, LEGUMES
  NUTS & SEEDS
  & ALTERNATIVES
  2 - 3 Servings Daily

- WHOLE GRAINS,
  CEREALS, PASTA &
  BROWN RICE
  3 - 4 Servings

- FRUITS
  (especially Apples
  & the skin)
  2 - 4 Servings Daily

- WATER
  8 Glasses Daily

8 Glasses Daily Purified/Distilled Water

22

Remember, LIVE FOODS produce healthy, LIVE PEOPLE!

PURIFIED WATER: Is at the pyramid's foundation. We recommend drinking *pure distilled water or any reliable, pure untreated water, free of toxins and chemicals* (pages 43-50). *Drink at least eight – 8 oz glasses of distilled water daily* and more if your lifestyle (like sports) requires it.

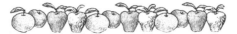

What a person eats and drinks becomes his own body chemistry.
– Dr. Paul C. Bragg

WHOLE GRAINS: Whole grains are the next pyramid level. **Avoid GMO processed, refined grain products (page 29)** and eat only unrefined, organic whole grain bread and cereals. Grains such as whole wheat, brown rice, oats, millet, quinoa, and 100% whole grain breads and cereals are best. One serving of whole grains is equal to 1 slice whole grain bread, 1 ounce ready-to-eat whole grain cereal, 1 cup cooked whole grains such as brown rice, oatmeal or other grains, 1 cup whole wheat, rice, pasta or noodles, and 1 ounce of other whole grain products. *We recommend eating 3 to 4 servings of whole grains a day.* This is because it is challenging to find truly GMO-free wheat in America. Many people of all ages discover they are gluten-sensitive. The wheat of today is not the wheat our grandparents consumed (see page 29). Gluten-free grains such as rice, buckwheat and quinoa are easier to digest and create less mucus as well.

VEGETABLES: We recommend eating as many of your vegetables organic and raw (uncooked, in salads, juices, smoothies, etc.) as possible! When cooking vegetables, do not overcook them. Steaming or lightly stir-frying is best. Vegetable juices also provide phytonutrients, vitamins and minerals. **The more colorful rainbow of vegetables you eat, the better they are for your health as they contain more valuable nutrients and healthy phytochemicals (page 35).** Eat a wide variety of organic vegetables daily. One vegetable serving is equal to 1 cup cooked vegetables or 1 cup raw uncooked vegetables, 1 cup salad, 3/4 cup vegetable juice. *We recommend 6 to 8 or more vegetable servings daily.*

FRUITS: Like vegetables, the more colorful the fruits the more healthy for you! Enjoy organic fruits as often as possible! One serving of fruit is equal to 1 medium apple, banana, orange, pear or other fruit, 1/2 cup fruit, 1/2 cup of fruit juice or 1/4 cup dried fruit. *We recommend eating 1 to 2 servings of organic fruits daily.*

Seek out, and choose healthy whole foods: organic fruits, vegetables, rice, beans, nuts and seeds, rather than the commercial, refined white flour and sugar products and highly processed canned goods in the center aisles.

The Bragg Healthy Lifestyle helps make a Healthier You and a Healthier World.

CALCIUM FOODS: Plant sources of calcium are healthier than dairy products because they don't contain saturated fats or cholesterol. Healthy plant-based calcium-rich foods are: Black-eyed peas, sesame seeds, almond milk, broccoli and green leafy vegetables (like kale and turnip greens). Serving sizes of plant-derived calcium-rich foods include: $^1/_2$ cup tofu, $^1/_3$ cup almonds, 1 cup cooked or 2 cups of high calcium raw greens, 1 cup of calcium-rich beans (white, navy, Great Northern), $^1/_2$ cup seaweed, 1 tablespoon blackstrap molasses, and 5 or more figs. *We recommend having 4 to 6 servings of healthy non-dairy sources of calcium rich foods daily.*

BEANS & LEGUMES: are healthy protein foods. Vegetable protein foods are more optimal compared to animal protein foods (plant-based protein chart on page 32). If you choose to eat animal protein, make sure it's organic, antibiotic- and hormone-free, and the fish is wild-caught, not farmed. Quality is of the utmost importance when it comes to animal protein in the diet. Vegetable proteins do not contain artery clogging saturated fats and cholesterol found in animal foods. They also contain protective factors to prevent heart disease, cancer and diabetes. Vegetable proteins provide the body with the essential amino acids that it requires. One serving of vegetable protein foods include: 1 cup cooked legumes (beans, lentils, dried peas), $^1/_2$ cup firm tofu or tempeh, 1 serving of "veggie meat" alternative veggieburger patty, 3 Tbsps. nut or seed butter, 1 cup almond or rice milk. *We recommend 2 to 3 or more vegetable protein servings daily.*

ESSENTIAL NUTRIENTS: are essential and healthy fats, like Omega-3's, vitamin D3 and minerals. Servings of healthy fats include: 1 tsp. of flaxseed oil, 1 Tbsp. of organic extra virgin olive oil, 3 tsps. of raw walnuts or pumpkin seeds. Other healthy essential nutrients include: ground flaxseeds or chia seeds and nutritional B-Complex supplements that provide vitamin B12. Do provide your body with the nutritional supplements your body requires for optimal health and longevity!

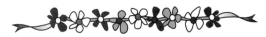

The secret of longevity is eating intelligently. – Gaylord Hauser

Healthy Foods Build & Maintain Your Body!

The person you are today, tomorrow, next week, next month and 10 years from now depends on what you eat! You are the sum total of the food you consume. How you look, feel and carry your years all depends on what you eat! Every part of your body is made from food – the hair on your head, your eyes, teeth, bones, blood and flesh. Even your expression is formed from what you eat, because the healthy man is a well-fed, happy man. We often jokingly say, "What are we going to feed our faces?" when it is plain that we mean our entire bodies (including our faces) are ready for nourishment.

We can begin anywhere in the body, but it's best starting with the skeleton which supports all other tissues. Superficially, our bones are largely minerals – mostly calcium and phosphate. One might suppose that once the skeleton is formed, nutrition of the bone stops. This is far from true! Using "isotopic tracers", top biochemists have found that, even in an adult body, minerals are constantly leaving and entering the bones. This means that bones are alive and are dynamic rather than static. Bones contain living cells which require not only minerals for building bone, but all the other food nutrients that living cells need to remain healthy! An emergency need for these cells arises when a bone is broken. If these cells had ceased to live and function when the adult skeleton became formed, a broken bone would remain broken for the rest of one's life. When a bone is broken, nourishment of these cells is crucially important! They not only need the minerals required for repairing the damage, but the cells themselves need to "eat" and keep healthy! These bone cells, like all other cells, can be nourished at various levels of efficiency. This is related to the fact that bones sometimes knit slowly and sometimes rapidly! The rate of healing can be slowed dramatically by poor nutrition of the cells, or it can be stepped up by improving the cell's nutrition!

When recovering from accidents, fractures, etc. it's important to take extra herbs, mineral and vitamin supplements to nourish and help your body heal faster! – Linda Page, N.D., Ph.D., author, "Healthy Healing" – See web: HealthyHealing.com

It's Important to Demand Healthy Foods

It is well worth the time and effort to read food labels – discard dead foods, and insist on fresh, live foods from reliable sources. We traveled around the world for our Bragg Health Crusades, and always found enough fresh, natural foods to maintain our Bragg Live Foods Lifestyle. If you know what to look for, ask around and you can find it. What the consumer strongly demands, long enough and loudly enough, the market supplies! Today (probably because so many people have health problems), there is a growing awareness on the importance of healthy nutrition. Today an increasing amount of supermarkets have health sections, and many have organic produce sections as well.

Watch Out for Hidden Sugars in Food Products

"Food labelers often hide sugars in their products by calling them by other names. They also use more than one kind of sugar, so that sugar will not have to be listed first, as the most common ingredient. In a list of ingredients, sugar can often be called: corn syrup, corn sweetener, high fructose corn syrup, dextrose, fructose, glucose, sorbitol, mannitol, barley malt, grape sweetener, sorghum, lactose and maltose. If even two of these "hidden" sugars are listed as the third and fourth ingredients, it may be that sugar is actually the highest ingredient in the product."
– *Healthy Heart Handbook*, Dr. Neal Pinckney

Sugar is Slow Suicide – Can Lead to Serious Diseases

High sugar consumption can overstimulate and harm your whole body system. Research Studies revealed one of the biggest hidden threats to health is consumption of all forms of sugar, which can lead to many serious health problems, ranging from: obesity, cancer, and heart trouble, to high blood sugar levels and diabetes.
– Dr. David Williams, *Mayo Clinic Guide to Healthy Living*

Sugar may increase the risk of tumor growth. Researchers found that a high amount of dietary sugar may increase the risk of tumor growth and cancer. Also too much refined sugar has been linked to obesity, Type 2 Diabetes, cardiovascular disease, and even dementia. The World Health Organization recommends that a daily intake of added sugars be below 5% or 6 tsps. The average American consumes 120 pounds of added sugar yearly!

Beware of Toxic, Deadly Aspartame and Chemical Sugar Substitutes!

Although its name sounds "tame," this deadly neurotoxin is anything but! Aspartame is an artificial sweetener (over 200 times sweeter than sugar) made by Monsanto Corporation and marketed as "Nutrasweet," "Equal," "Spoonful," and countless other trade names. Although aspartame is added to over 9,000 food products, it is not fit for human consumption! This toxic poison changes into formaldehyde in the body and has been linked to migraines, seizures, vision loss and symptoms relating to Lupus, Parkinson's Disease, Multiple Sclerosis and other health destroying conditions! Besides being a deadly poison, aspartame actually contributes to weight gain by causing a craving for carbohydrates! A study of 80,000 women by the American Cancer Society found those who used this toxic "diet" sweetener actually gained more weight than those who didn't use aspartame products. To learn more about the deadly health risks and crime against our precious health, check web: *usrtk.org/sweeteners/aspartame_health_risks/*

High Fructose Corn Syrup (HFCS), is a highly toxic processed sugar that contains similar amounts of unbound fructose and glucose. What makes HFCS unhealthy is that it is metabolized to fat in your body far more rapidly than any other sugar. It is a primary factor behind a number of health epidemics, including obesity, diabetes and heart disease. For a better sugar substitute use herb Stevia.

STEVIA – A Natural Herbal Sweetener

Stevia – the natural herbal sweetener is an herb native to South America. It is widely grown for its sweet leaves. In its unprocessed form it is 30 times sweeter than sugar. It is a low carbohydrate, low-sugar food alternative. Stevia shows promise for treating such conditions as obesity and high blood pressure. It does not effect blood sugar and it even enhances glucose tolerance. It helps mental alertness, combats fatigue and improves digestion. Stevia is calorie-free and a safe, delicious, health sweetener for diabetics. Children can use Stevia without concerns, as it does not cause cavities. Look for 100% pure stevia with no additives when shopping
See web: stevia.com

White Sugar Destroys Teeth, Bones & Health

The American fast, junk food diet, in addition to lacking vitamins and minerals, is also highly acid-producing, due to the high proportion of refined white sugar, white flour and animal proteins, which increase acidity of the body with adverse effects on bones and health. Strong bones require an alkaline balance within the body metabolism, naturally maintained by a higher proportion of raw organic fruits and vegetables in the diet. The worst villain is refined white sugar and its many products; there is no single food more devastating to the spine and other bones of the body. Sugar leaches calcium, phosphorus, magnesium and manganese out of the bones, making them weak, porous and brittle! Candy, sweets, refined white sugar products and all sugared drinks are prime causes of tooth decay and diabetes. Since teeth are the body's hardest tissue, you can understand what refined white sugar does to other bones and cartilages (protective cushions between bones) of the skeletal system, including the spinal column. *(HealingDaily.com/detoxification-diet/sugar.htm)*

28

Bad Nutrition is #1 Cause of Sickness

"Diet-related diseases account for 68% of all Americans' deaths."
– Dr. C. Everett Koop

America's former top Surgeon General and our friend, said this in his famous 1988 Landmark Report on Nutrition and Health in America. People don't die of infectious conditions as such, but of malnutrition

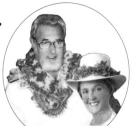

Dr. Koop & Patricia
Hawaii Health Conference

that allows the germs to get a foothold in sickly bodies. Also, bad nutrition is usually the cause of non-infectious, fatal or degenerative conditions. When the body has its full nutrition quota of vitamins and minerals, including potassium, it's almost impossible for germs to get a foothold in a healthy, powerful bloodstream and tissues!

"Paul Bragg did more for the Health of America than any one person I know of." – Former US Surgeon General, C. Everett Koop

Beware: Why "Modern" Wheat is Bad for You

"Modern wheat isn't really wheat at all and is a *perfect, chronic poison,*" according to Dr. William Davis, a Cardiologist, author and leading expert on wheat, the world's most popular grain. *Dr. Davis explains that "the wheat we eat today (even though it may say 100% whole wheat), isn't the wheat your ancestors had, it's an 18" tall plant created by genetic research in the 60's and 70's. There's a new protein in this type of wheat called Gliadin, which is an opiate. Gliadin binds into opiate receptors in the brain and in most people stimulates the appetite then they eat more food daily and become obese!

Modern wheat is responsible for eight out of ten people's health problems. Researchers have found that once wheat is removed from their diet, their illnesses disappeared within three to six months. People who turn away from wheat have dropped substantial weight. Even diabetics no longer become diabetic; people with arthritis have dramatic relief. Along with less acid reflux; leg swelling; irritable bowel syndrome, as well as depression.

So why is modern wheat bad? Wheat is one of the oldest known grains. On a cellular level, our bodies simply don't recognize this new species of grain. Some people's bodies simply have a hard time digesting it leading to gas, constipation and diarrhea. Others have 'brain fog' dizziness, inflammation and migraines.

As with other commercially grown grains, scientists began cross-breeding wheat plants to arrive at new varieties that are hardier, shorter, and yield more. In fact, the newer, high-yield hybridized wheat we've been eating since the 1980's has been selectively bred to produce high gluten grains that seem to trigger inflammatory responses in our body, causing more problems than ever! Among the diseases attributed to the consumption of wheat is Celiac disease."

Dr. Davis goes on to say, "that there is no nutrient deficiency that develops when eliminating wheat from your diet. Replace wheat with organic healthy foods like vegetables, nuts, avocados. Try eliminating grains, that's when you'll see transformations in your health." (*Web: *IntentionalWellnessInc.com/nutrition/wheat-is-bad-for-you*)

Food and Product Summary

Today, many of our foods are highly processed or refined, robbing them of essential nutrients, vitamins, minerals and enzymes. Many also contain harmful, toxic and dangerous GMO chemicals. Research findings and experience of top nutritionists, physicians and dentists have led to the discovery that devitalized foods are a major cause of poor health, illness, cancer and premature death! The enormous increase in the last 70 years of degenerative diseases such as heart disease, arthritis, diabetes and dental decay, etc. back this belief. Scientific research shows most of these afflictions can be prevented and others, once established, can be arrested or even reversed through nutritional methods.

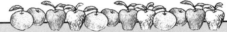

Enjoy Super Health with Natural Foods

1. **RAW FOODS:** Fresh fruits and raw vegetables organically grown are always best! Enjoy nutritious variety garden salads with raw vegetables, sprouts, raw nuts and seeds.

2. **VEGETABLES and PROTEINS:**
   a. Legumes, lentils, brown rice and all beans.
   b. Nuts and seeds, raw and unsalted (lightly roasted okay).
   c. We prefer healthier vegetarian proteins. If you must have animal protein, then be sure it's hormone-free, and organically fed and no more than 1 or 2 times a week.
   d. Dairy products – fertile range-free eggs (four weekly), unprocessed hard cheese and feta goat's cheese. We choose not to use dairy products. Try the healthier non-dairy rice, coconut, oat and almond milks

3. **FRUITS and VEGETABLES:** Organically grown is always best – grown without the use of poisonous sprays and toxic chemical fertilizers whenever possible; do urge your markets to stock healthier organic produce! Steam, bake, sauté and wok vegetables as short a time as possible to retain the best nutritional content and flavor. Also enjoy fresh juices.

4. **ORGANIC non-GMO WHOLE GRAINS, CEREALS, BREADS:** Barley, rye, buckwheat, spelt, teff, oatmeal, quinoa, millet, amaranth, wild rice, etc. contain important B-complex vitamins, vitamin E, minerals, fiber and unsaturated fatty acids.

5. **COLD or EXPELLER-PRESSED VEGETABLE OILS:** Organic, first press, extra virgin olive oil (is best), flax, sunflower, and sesame oils are good sources of healthy, essential, unsaturated fatty acids. We still use oils sparingly.

The Bragg Healthy Lifestyle Promotes Super Health & Longevity

The Bragg Healthy Lifestyle consists of eating a diet of 60% to 70% fresh, live, organically grown foods; raw vegetables, salads, fresh fruits and juices; sprouts, raw seeds and nuts; all-natural 100% whole-grain breads, pastas, cereals and nutritious beans and legumes. These are the no-cholesterol, no-fat, no-salt, "live foods" which combine to make up the body fuel that creates healthy, lively people that want to exercise and be fit. This is the reason people become revitalized and reborn into a fresh new life filled with joy, health, vitality, youthfulness and longevity! **We have millions of healthy followers around the world proving that The Bragg Healthy Lifestyle works miracles for them!** *Now it's your turn!*

Enjoy Healthy Fiber for Super Health

These are our suggestions for healthy fiber:

31

- **EAT ALL VARIETIES OF ORGANIC BERRIES,** surprisingly good sources of fiber.

- **KEEP BEANS HANDY,** probably the best fiber sources. Cook dried beans and freeze in portions. Use canned beans for faster meals.

- **INSTEAD OF ICEBERG LETTUCE,** choose deep green lettuces such as romaine, bib, butter, spinach or cabbage.

- **LOOK FOR "100% ORGANIC WHOLE WHEAT"** or whole grain breads, when eating bread.

- **LOOK FOR WHOLE GRAIN or RICE CEREALS.**

- **GO FOR BROWN RICE** over white rice.

- **EAT THE SKIN** of the potato, fruits and vegetables.

- **SERVE HUMMUS,** made from chickpeas, instead of sour-cream with your dip.

- **DON'T UNDERESTIMATE NON-GMO ORGANIC CORN,** especially popcorn and corn tortillas.

- **ADD ORGANIC OAT BRAN & WHEAT-GERM** to baked goods.

- **SNACK ON ORGANIC SUN-DRIED FRUIT.**

- **INSTEAD OF DRINKING FRUIT JUICE,** eat whole fruit.

The first requisite of a good life is to be a healthy person.
– Herbert Spencer

Plant-Based Protein Chart

BEANS & LEGUMES

(1 cup cooked)	PROTEIN IN GRAMS
Lentils	18
Adzuki Beans	17
Cannellini	17
Navy Beans	16
Split Peas	16
Black Beans	15
Garbanzos (chick peas)	15
Kidney Beans	15
Great Northern Beans	15
Lima Beans	15
Chick Peas	15
Black-eyed Peas	14
Pinto Beans	14
Mung Beans	14
Tofu (3 oz.)	7 to 12
Green Peas (whole)	9

RAW NUTS & SEEDS

(1/4 cup or 4 Tbsps)	PROTEIN IN GRAMS
Chia Seeds	12
Macadamia Nuts	11
Flax Seeds	8
Sunflower Seeds	8
Almonds	7
Pumpkin Seeds	7
Sesame Seeds	7
Walnuts	5
Brazil Nuts	5
Hazelnuts	5
Pine Nuts	4
Cashews	4

32

NUT BUTTERS

(2 Tbsps)	PROTEIN IN GRAMS
Peanut Butter	7 to 9
Almond Butter	5 to 8
Cashew Butter	4 to 5
Sesame - Tahini	6

VEGETABLES

(1 Serving or 1 cup)	PROTEIN IN GRAMS
Spirulina	8.6
Corn (1 cob)	5
Potato (with skin)	5
Mushrooms, Oyster	5
Artichoke (1 medium)	4
Collard Greens	4
Broccoli	4
Brussel Sprouts	4
Mushrooms, Shiitake	3.5
Swiss Chard	3
Kale	2.5
Asparagus (5 spears)	2
String Beans	2
Beets	2
Peas	2
Sweet Potato	3
Summer Squash	2
Cabbage	2
Carrot	2
Cauliflower	2
Squash	2
Celery	1
Spinach	1
Bell Peppers	1
Cucumber	1
Eggplant	1
Leeks	1
Lettuce	1
Tomato (1 medium)	1
Radish	1
Turnips	1

DAIRY & NUT MILKS

(1 cup)	PROTEIN IN GRAMS
Oat Milk	3
Almond Milk	1 to 2
Rice Milk	1
Eggs (1) *(free-range)*	6

FRUITS

(1 Serving or 1 cup)	PROTEIN IN GRAMS
Avocado (1 medium)	4
Banana (1)	1 to 2
Blackberries (1 cup)	2
Pomegranate (1)	1.5
Blueberries (1 cup)	1
Cantaloupe (1 cup)	1
Cherries (1 cup)	1
Grapes (1 cup)	1
Honeydew (1 cup)	1
Kiwi (1 large)	1
Lemon (1)	1
Mango (1)	1
Nectarine (1)	1
Orange (1)	1
Peach (1)	1
Pear (1)	1
Pineapple (1 cup)	1
Plum (1)	1
Raspberries (1 cup)	1
Strawberries (1 cup)	1
Watermelon (1 cup)	1

GRAINS & RICE

(1 cup cooked)	PROTEIN IN GRAMS
Triticale	25
Millet	8.4
Amaranth	7
Oat Bran	7
Wild Rice	7
Couscous (whole wheat)	6
Bulgur Wheat	6
Buckwheat	6
Teff	6
Oat Groats	6
Barley	5
Quinoa	5
Brown Rice	5
Spelt	5

This chart displays protein content of common vegetarian foods. Note that in order to determine amount of protein that is optimal for your body, use the following formula that is based on a vegan diet: *RDA recommends that we take in 0.36 grams of protein per pound that we weigh* (100 lbs. x 0.36 = 36 grams).

Data from webs: *TheHolyKale.com • VegParadise.com • vrg.org (Vegetarian Resource Group).*

What are Nature's Miracle Phytonutrients?

These wonderful, organic compounds are found in plants, (*phyto* means 'plant' in Greek), that are vital to human health. Increasingly, scientific studies are showing that phytonutrients help protect us from many serious health issues, including heart disease and stroke. Organic fruits, vegetables, grains, legumes, nuts, seeds and some teas are rich in the miracle phytonutrients.

Plants contain more than 10,000 phytonutrients, one reason 10-14 servings of fruits and veggies daily are recommended. Plants and vegetables contain different phytonutrients, so having a variety in diet is important.

Physicians and scientists have written about the critical nature of these foods for thousands of years, but the specific benefits of phytonutrients are still being discovered. They are created when plants absorb energy from the earth, water, air and sun. This energy helps plants survive environmental challenges such as diseases, injures, drought, excessive heat, ultraviolet sunrays and poisons. This incredible energy forms an important part of the plant's immune system! It appears to provide humans with the same benefits, when we consume the plants! They help increase our immune and regeneration systems. Plants give us strength, endurance, health and ultimately help us feel better and live longer.

Increasing fruits and vegetables in your diet can help prevent heart disease, cancer and other chronic diseases. Surveys show those who increased daily fruit and vegetables improved their health, vitality and well-being. – UC Berkeley Wellness Letter • BerkeleyWellness.com

Swapping beans, nuts, or veggie burgers for meat means you get fiber, which fills you up, aids digestion, and balances gut bacteria, and you up your intake of unsaturated fatty acids. These beneficial fats are found in foods like nuts and seeds, that support your brain and heart.

A nine year study showed that people who eat pears are less likely to be obese. Just a pear a day has high levels of vitamin C, fiber and offers protection against colon cancer and helps reduce blood LDL cholesterol levels.

Antioxidants & Phytonutrients Health Benefits

The body must have these important phytonutrients and enzymes to break food down, kill viruses and bacteria and dissolve tumors! A diet of at least 50% raw, unprocessed foods is vital to make sure that we are getting enough enzymes and phytonutrients to optimize the body's processes.

On average, plant foods have 64 times more antioxidants than animal foods, which is critical because when it comes to antioxidants, the more we eat, the more our heath benefits! Eating a diet high in antioxidants is important because they reduce inflammation and free radicals in the body and help protect against heart disease and cancer. See chart on the next page for health benefits of different plant sources. See web: *hsph.Harvard.edu/NutritionSource/antioxidants.*

Main Sources of Miracle Phytonutrients

The following are high in phytonutrients: carrots and yellow vegetables (sweet potatoes and pumpkins), peaches, apricots, broccoli, leafy greens (kale, spinach, turnip greens), tomatoes, pink grapefruit, watermelon, guava, apples, blackberries, walnuts, strawberries, cranberries, raspberries, blueberries, grape juice, prunes, red cabbage, pomegranates, pineapple, oranges, plums, pinto beans, kiwi fruit and red chile peppers.

The more live, unprocessed foods we eat the more phytonutrients and enzymes we consume the healthier our diet. This natural food is full of the energy we need to live healthier, longer lives! To boost your immune system and cell regeneration eat more phytonutrients, practice deep breathing exercises daily, get physical exercise, and make sure your diet is at least 50-60% raw, healthy, organic foods! That's *The Bragg Healthy Lifestyle* and when followed produces miracles.

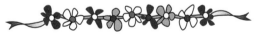

Life cannot be maintained unless life be taken in. And this is best done by making at least 50-60% of your diet raw and with a plentiful supply of fresh juicy organic fruits and some lightly cooked vegetables.
– Patricia Bragg, Pioneer Health Crusader

Mother Nature's Miracle Phytonutrients Help Prevent Cancer

Make sure to get your daily dose of naturally occurring, cancer-fighting super foods – Phytonutrients are abundant in apples, tomatoes, onions, garlic, beans, legumes, soybeans, cabbage, cauliflower, broccoli, citrus, etc. Champions with highest count of Phytonutrients – apples and tomatoes.

Phytonutrient	Food Sources	Health Action
PHYTOESTROGEN ISOFLAVONES	Soy products, flaxseed, seeds and nuts, yams, alfalfa, pomegranates lentils, carrots, apples	Helps block some cancers, aids in menopausal symptoms, balances hormones, helps improve memory, enhances heart health
PHYTOSTEROLS	Plant oils: corn, sesame, safflower; rice bran, wheat germ, peanuts	Blocks hormonal role in cancers, inhibits uptake of cholesterol from diet, reduce risk of heart attack
LIGNANS	Flaxseeds, rye, lentils, soy mushrooms, barley	Helps prevent breast cancer, heart disease and balances hormones
SAPONINS	Yams, beets, beans, cabbage, nuts, soybeans	Helps prevent cancer cells from multiplying, reduces cholesterol
TERPENES	Carrots, winter squash, sweet potatoes, yams, apples, cantaloupes, cherries	Antioxidants – protects DNA from free radical-induced damage, and improves immunity
	Tomatoes and its sauces, tomato-based products	Helps block UVA & UVB and offers help to protect against cancers – breast, prostate, etc.
	Spinach, kale, beet and turnip greens, cabbage	Protects eyes from macular degeneration,
	Red chile peppers	Keeps carcinogens from binding to DNA
QUERCETIN (& FLAVONOIDS)	Apples (especially the skins), red onions and green tea	Strong cancer fighter, protects heart - arteries. Reduces pain, allergy and asthma symptoms
	Citrus fruits (flavonoids)	Promotes protective enzymes
PHENOLS	Apples, fennel, parsley, carrots, alfalfa, cabbage	Helps prevent blood clotting & has important anticancer properties
	Cinnamon	Promotes healthy blood sugar and glucose metabolism
	Citrus fruits, broccoli, cabbage, cucumbers, green peppers, tomatoes	Antioxidants – flavonoids, block membrane receptor sites for certain hormones
	Apples, grape seeds	Strong antioxidants; fights germs and bacteria, strengthens immune system, veins and capillaries
	Grapes, especially skins	Antioxidant, antimutagen; promotes detoxification. Acts as carcinogen inhibitors
	Yellow and green squash	Antihepatotoxic, antitumor
SULFUR COMPOUNDS	Onions and garlic, (fresh is always best) Red onions (our favorite) also contain Quercetin Onions help keep doctor away	Promotes liver enzymes, inhibits cholesterol synthesis, reduces triglycerides, lowers blood pressure improves immune response, fights infections, germs and parasites

35

Paul C. Bragg Introduced Juicing to America

Juicing has come a long way since the first hand operated vegetable-fruit juicers from Europe were available. Before, this juice was pressed by hand using cheesecloth. He introduced his new juice therapy idea, then pineapple juice, then later tomato juice, to the American public. These two juices were erroneously thought to be too acidic. Now, these health beverages have become the favorites of millions. TV's famous *Juicemen* Jay Kordich and Jack LaLanne say Paul Bragg was their early inspiration and mentor! LaLanne also has a great juicer. They both loved living The Bragg Healthy Lifestyle and inspiring millions to health.

Delicious Juice / Blender Combinations:

1. Beet, celery, alfalfa sprouts
2. Cabbage, celery and apple
3. Cabbage, cucumber, celery, tomato, spinach and basil
4. Tomato, carrot and celery
5. Carrot, celery, watercress, apple, garlic and wheatgrass
6. Grapefruit, orange and lemon
7. Beet, parsley, celery, carrot, mustard greens, cabbage, garlic
8. Beet, celery, kelp and carrot
9. Cucumber, carrot and celery
10. Watercress, apple, cucumber, garlic
11. Asparagus, carrot and celery
12. Carrot, celery, parsley and cabbage, onion, sweet basil
13. Carrot, coconut milk and ginger
14. Carrot, broccoli, lemon, cayenne
15. Carrot, sprouts, kelp, rosemary
16. Apple, carrot, radish, ginger
17. Apple, pineapple and ginger
18. Apple, papaya and grapes
19. Papaya, cranberries and apple
20. Leafy greens, broccoli, apple
21. Grape, apple and blueberries
22. Watermelon (alone is best)

Liquefy or Juice Fresh Organic Fruits & Veggies

The juicer, food processor and blender are great for preparing foods, drinks, gentle (bland) diets and baby foods. Fibers of juiced fresh fruits and vegetables can be tolerated on most gentle diets. Any raw or cooked fruit or vegetable can be liquefied and added to broth, soups and non-dairy (soy, rice or nut) milks. Fresh juices supercharge your energy level and boost your immune system to maximize your body's health power. You may fortify liquid meals or Bragg Smoothies with any green vegetable powders, alfalfa, barley green, chlorella, spirulina and wheat grass for extra nutrition.

BENEFITS FROM THE JOYS OF FASTING

Fasting renews your faith in yourself, your strength and God's strength.
Fasting is easier than any diet.
Fasting is the quickest way to lose weight.
Fasting is adaptable to a busy life.
Fasting gives the body a physiological rest.
Fasting is used successfully in the treatment of many physical illnesses.
Fasting can yield weight losses of up to 10 pounds or more in the first week.
Fasting lowers and normalizes cholesterol, homocysteine, blood pressure levels.
Fasting improves dietary habits.
Fasting increases pleasure eating healthy foods.
Fasting is a calming experience, often relieving tension and insomnia.
Fasting frequently induces feelings of happy euphoria, a natural high.
Fasting is a miracle rejuvenator, helps in slowing the ageing process.
Fasting is a natural stimulant to rejuvenate the growth hormone levels.
Fasting is an energizer, not a debilitator.
Fasting aids the elimination process.
Fasting often results in a more vigorous happy marital relationship.
Fasting can eliminate smoking, drug and drinking addictions.
Fasting is a regulator, educating the body to consume food only as needed.
Fasting saves precious time spent on marketing, preparing and eating.
Fasting rids the body of toxins, giving it an internal shower and cleansing.
Fasting does not deprive the body of essential nutrients.
Fasting can be used to uncover the sources of food allergies.
Fasting is used effectively in schizophrenia and other mental illness treatment.
Fasting under proper supervision can be tolerated easily up to four weeks.
Fasting does not accumulate appetite; hunger pangs disappear in 1-2 days.
Fasting is routine for most of the animal kingdom.
Fasting has been a common practice since the beginning of man's existence.
Fasting is practiced in all religions; the Bible alone has 74 references to fasting.
Fasting under proper conditions is absolutely safe.
Fasting is a blessing – "Fasting As A Way Of Life" – Allan Cott, M.D.
Fasting is not starving, it's nature's cure that God has given us. – Patricia Bragg

Dear Health Friend,

This gentle reminder explains the great benefits from "The Miracle of Fasting" that you will enjoy when starting on your weekly 24-hour Bragg Fasting Program for Super Health! It's a precious time of body-mind-soul cleansing and renewal.

On fast days I drink 8-10 glasses of distilled (our favorite) or purified water, (I add 1-2 tsps. organic apple cider vinegar to three of them). If just starting, you may also try herbal teas or try diluted fresh juices with 1/3 distilled water. Every day, even on fast days, add 1 Tbsp. of psyllium husk powder to liquids once daily. It's an extra cleanser and helps normalize weight, cholesterol and blood pressure and helps promote healthy elimination. Fasting is the oldest, most effective healing method known to man. Fasting offers great miraculous blessings from Mother Nature and our Creator. It begins the self-cleansing of the inner-body workings so we can promote our own self-healing.

My father and I wrote the book "The Miracle of Fasting" to share with you the health miracles it can perform in your life. It's all so worthwhile to do. It's an important part of The Bragg Healthy Lifestyle.

With Love,

Patricia

Paul Bragg's work on fasting and water is one of the great contributions to The Healing Wisdom and The Natural Health Movement in the world today.
– Gabriel Cousens, M.D., author "Conscious Eating" and "Spiritual Nutrition"

37

Avoid These Processed, Refined, Harmful Foods:

Once you realize the harm caused to your body by unhealthy refined, chemicalized, deficient foods, you'll want to eliminate "killer" foods:

- **Refined sugar / artificial sweeteners** (toxic aspartame) or their products such as jams, jellies, preserves, marmalades, yogurts, ice cream, sherbets, Jello, cake, candy, cookies, all chewing gum, colas and diet drinks, pies, pastries, and all sugared fruit juices and fruits canned in sugar syrup. (Health Stores have delicious healthy replacements, such as Stevia, raw honey, 100% maple syrup, and monk fruit, so seek and buy the best).

- **White flour products** such as white bread, wheat-white bread, enriched flours, rye bread that has white flour in it, dumplings, biscuits, buns, gravy, pasta, pancakes, waffles, soda crackers, pizza, ravioli, pies, pastries, cakes, cookies, prepared and commercial puddings and ready-mix bakery products. Most are made with dangerous (oxy-cholesterol) powdered milk and powdered eggs. (Health Stores have a variety of 100% non-GMO whole grain organic products, breads, chips, crackers, pastas, desserts).

- **Salted foods,** such as pretzels, corn chips, potato chips, crackers and nuts.

- **Refined white rice** and pearl barley. • **Fried fast foods.** • **Indian ghee**.

- **Refined dry processed cereals** that are sugared, such as cornflakes, etc.

- **Foods that contain Olestra,** palm and cottonseed oil.

- **Peanuts and peanut butter** that contain hydrogenated, hardened oils and any peanuts with mold and all molds that can cause allergies.

- **Margarine** – combines heart-deadly trans-fatty acids and saturated fats.

- **Saturated fats and hydrogenated oils** – enemies that clog the arteries.

- **Coffee, soft drinks, teas, alcohol, sugared juices** – even if decaffeinated.

- **Fresh pork / products.** • **Fried, fatty, greasy meats.** • **Irradiated GMO foods.**

- **Smoked meats,** such as ham, bacon, sausage and all smoked fish.

- **Luncheon meats,** hot dogs, salami, bologna, corned beef, pastrami and packaged meats containing dangerous sodium nitrate or nitrite.

- **Dried fruits** containing sulphur dioxide – a toxic preservative.

- **Chickens, turkeys and meats injected with hormones** or fed with commercial feed containing any drugs or toxins.

- **Canned soups** – read labels for sugar, salt, starch, flour and preservatives.

- **Foods containing preservatives, additives,** benzoate of soda, salt, sugar, cream of tartar, drugs, irradiated and genetically engineered foods.

- **Day-old cooked vegetables,** potatoes and pre-mixed, wilted lifeless salads.

- **All commercial vinegars:** pasteurized, filtered, distilled, white, malt and synthetic vinegars are dead vinegars! (We use only unfiltered Apple Cider Vinegar with "Mother Enzyme" as used in olden times.)

Please follow The Bragg Healthy Lifestyle to provide the basic, healthy nourishment to maintain your precious health.

Allergies & Dr. Coca's Pulse Test

Almost every known food may cause some allergic reaction at times. Thus, foods used in *elimination* diets may cause allergic reactions in some individuals. Some are listed among the *Most Common Food Allergies* (see below). Since reaction to these foods is generally low, they are widely used in making test diets. By keeping a food journal and tracking your pulse rate after meals you will soon know your *problem* foods. Allergic foods cause pulse to then go up. (Take base pulse, for 1 minute, before meals, then 30 minutes after meals, and also before bed. If it increases 8-10 beats per minute – check foods for allergies.)

If your body has a reaction after eating some particular food, especially if it happens each time you eat that food, you may have an allergy. Some allergic reactions are: wheezing, sneezing, stuffy nose, nasal drip or mucus, dark circles, eye watering or bags under your eyes, headaches, feeling light-headed or dizzy, fast heart beat, stomach or chest pains, diarrhea, extreme thirst, breaking out in a rash, swelling of extremities or stomach bloating, etc. (read Dr. Arthur Coca's book, *The Pulse Test*.)

If you know what you're allergic to, you are lucky; if you don't, you had better find out as fast as possible and eliminate all irritating foods from your diet. To re-evaluate your daily life and have a health guide to your future, start a daily journal (copy page 42) of foods eaten, your pulse rate before and after meals and your reactions, moods, energy levels, weight, elimination and sleep patterns. You will discover the foods and situations causing problems. **By charting your diet you will be amazed at the effects of eating certain foods. We have kept daily journals for years.**

If you are hypersensitive to certain foods, you must omit them from your diet! There are hundreds of allergies and of course it's impossible here to take up each one. Many have allergies to milk, wheat, or some are allergic to all grains. **Visit web: *FoodAllergy.org*. Your daily journal will help you discover and accurately pinpoint the foods and situations causing you problems. Start your journal today!**

Most Common Food Allergies

- **DAIRY:** butter, cheese, cottage cheese, ice cream, milk, yogurt, etc.
- **CEREALS & GRAINS:** wheat, corn, buckwheat, oats, rye, triticale (gluten)
- **EGGS:** cakes, custards, dressings, mayonnaise, noodles
- **FISH:** shellfish, crabs, lobster, shrimp, shad roe
- **MEATS:** bacon, beef, chicken, pork, sausage, veal, smoked products
- **FRUITS:** citrus fruits, melons, strawberries
- **NUTS:** peanuts, pecans, walnuts, chemically dried preserved nuts
- **ALL ARTIFICIAL:** colors and preservatives, dyes and chemicals
- **MISCELLANEOUS:** chocolate, cocoa, coffee, black and green teas, palm and cottonseed oils, MSG, salt. Also, allergic reactions are often caused by toxic pesticides or sprays on salad greens, vegetables and fruits.

HEALTHY BEVERAGES
Fresh Juices, Herb Teas & Energy Drinks

These freshly squeezed organic vegetable and fruit juices are important to *The Bragg Healthy Lifestyle*. It's not wise to drink beverages with your main meals, as it dilutes the digestive juices. But it's great during the day to have a glass of freshly squeezed orange juice, grapefruit juice, vegetable juice, raw, organic apple cider vinegar drink (see below), or herbal tea – these are all ideal pick-me-up beverages.

Apple Cider Vinegar Drink – Mix 1-2 tsps. raw, organic apple cider vinegar (with the 'Mother' enzyme) and (optional) to taste raw honey or pure maple syrup *(if diabetic, to sweeten use 2 stevia drops)* in 8 oz. of distilled or purified water. Take glass upon arising, an hour before lunch and dinner.

Delicious Hot or Cold Cider Drink – Add 2-3 cinnamon sticks and 4 cloves to water and boil. Steep 20 minutes or more. Before serving add raw organic apple cider vinegar and sweetener to taste.

Bragg's Favorite Juice Drink – This drink consists of all raw vegetables *(remember organic is best)* which we prepare in our juicer / blender: carrots, celery, cucumber, beets, cabbage, tomatoes, watercress, kale, parsley, or any vegetable combination you prefer. The great purifier, garlic we enjoy, but it's optional.

Bragg's Favorite Healthy Energy Smoothie – After our morning stretch and exercises we often enjoy this drink instead of fruit. It's a delicious and powerfully nutritious meal anytime: lunch, dinner or in a thermos at work, school, the gym or during sports or hikes. You can freeze for popsicles too.

Bragg's Favorite Healthy Energy Smoothie

Prepare the following in a blender, add frozen juice cubes if desired colder; Choice of: freshly squeezed orange or grapefruit juice; carrot and greens juice; unsweetened pineapple juice; or $1^1/2$ - 2 cups purified or distilled water with:

2 tsps spirulina or green powder
$1/3$ tsp nutritional yeast
2 dates or prunes-pitted
1 "Emergen-C" Vitamin C packet
1 tsp protein powder (optional)

1-2 bananas or fresh fruit
1-2 tsps almond or nut butter
1 tsp flaxseed oil or grind seeds
1 tsp raw honey (optional)
$1/2$ tsp lecithin granules

Optional: 4-6 apricots (sun-dried) soak in jar overnight in purified distilled water or unsweetened pineapple juice. We soak enough to last for several days. Keep refrigerated. In summer you can add organic fresh fruit: peaches, papaya, blueberries, strawberries, all berries, apricots, instead of banana. In winter, add apples, kiwi, oranges, tangelos, persimmons or pears, and if fresh is unavailable, try sugar-free, frozen organic fruits. Serves 1 to 2.

Patricia's Delicious Health Popcorn

Use freshly popped organic popcorn (use air popper). Drizzle organic olive oil, melted coconut oil or salt-free butter over popcorn. Sprinkle with good quality nutritional yeast for amazing flavor. For a variety try a pinch of cayenne pepper, mustard powder or fresh crushed garlic to oil mixture. Serve instead of breads!

Nutrition directly affects growth, development, reproduction, well-being of an individual's physical and mental condition. Health depends upon nutrition more than on any other single factor. – Dr. William H. Sebrell, Jr.

Lentil & Brown Rice Casserole, Burgers or Soup
Paul Bragg and Jack LaLanne's Favorite Recipe

16 oz pkg organic lentils, uncooked
1 cup brown organic rice, uncooked
5 cups, distilled / purified water
4-6 carrots, chop $^1/2"$ rounds
3 celery stalks, chop

4 garlic cloves, chop
2 onions, chop
2 tsps organic coconut aminos
1 tsp salt-free all-purpose seasoning
2 tsps organic extra-virgin olive oil

1 cup diced fresh or canned tomatoes (salt-free)

Wash and drain lentils and rice. Place grains in large stainless steel pot. Add water, bring to boil, reduce heat and simmer 30 minutes. Now add vegetables and seasonings and cook on low heat until tender. Last five minutes add fresh or canned (salt-free) tomatoes. For delicious garnish, add minced parsley & nutritional yeast. **For Burgers mash. For Soup, add more water in cooking grains.** Serves 4 to 6.

Raw Organic Vegetable Health Salad

2 stalks celery, chop
1 bell pepper & seeds, dice
$^1/2$ cucumber, slice
2 carrots, grate
1 raw beet, grate
1 cup green cabbage, chop

$^1/2$ cup red cabbage, chop
$^1/2$ cup alfalfa, mung or sunflower sprouts
2 spring onions & green tops, chop
1 turnip, grate
1 avocado (ripe)
3 tomatoes, medium size

For variety add organic raw zucchini, peas, mushrooms, broccoli, cauliflower, (try black olives and pasta). Chop, slice or grate vegetables fine to medium for variety in size. Mix vegetables & serve on bed of lettuce, spinach, chopped kale or cabbage. Dice avocado and tomato and serve on side as a dressing. Serve choice of fresh squeezed lemon, orange or dressing separately. Chill salad plates before serving. **It's best to always eat salad first before hot dishes.** Serves 3 to 5.

41

Patricia's Health Salad Dressing

$^1/2$ cup raw organic apple cider vinegar
1-2 tsps organic raw honey

$^1/2$ tsp organic coconut aminos
1-2 cloves garlic, minced

$^1/3$ cup organic extra-virgin olive oil, or blend with safflower, sesame or flax oil
1 Tbsp fresh herbs, minced (to taste)

Blend ingredients in blender or jar. Refrigerate in covered jar.

For delicious Herbal Vinegar: In quart jar add $^1/3$ cup tightly packed, crushed fresh sweet basil, tarragon, dill, oregano, or any fresh herbs desired, combined or singly (if dried herbs, use 1-2 tsps herbs). Now cover to top with raw, organic apple cider vinegar and store two weeks in warm place, and then strain and refrigerate.

Honey – Chia or Celery Seed Vinaigrette

$^1/4$ tsp dry mustard
$^1/4$ tsp organic coconut aminos
$^1/4$ tsp paprika or to taste
1-2 Tbsps honey

1 cup organic apple cider vinegar
$^1/2$ cup organic extra-virgin olive oil
$^1/2$ small onion, minced
$^1/3$ tsp chia or celery seed (or vary to taste)

Blend ingredients in blender or jar. Refrigerate in covered jar.

Studies show both beta carotene and vitamin C, abundantly found in fruits and vegetables, play vital roles in preventing heart disease and cancers.

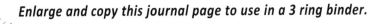
Enlarge and copy this journal page to use in a 3 ring binder.

MY DAILY HEALTH JOURNAL

Today is:___/___/___

> *I have said my morning resolve and am ready to practice faithfully The Bragg Healthy Lifestyle today and every day.*

Yesterday I went to bed at: Today I arose at: Weight:

Today I practiced the No-Heavy Breakfast or No-Breakfast Plan: ☐ yes ☐ no

- For Breakfast I drank: Time:

  For Breakfast I ate:
              Time:

  Supplements:

- For Lunch I ate: Time:

  Supplements:

- For Dinner I ate: Time:

  Supplements:

- ____ Glasses of Water I Drank during the Day, including ACV Drinks

  List Snacks – Type and When:

_____

- I took part in these physical activities (walking, gym, etc.) today:

_____

Grade each on scale of 1 to 10 (desired optimum health is 10).
- I rate my day for the following categories:

  Previous Night's Sleep: Stress/Anxiety:

  Energy Level: Elimination:

  Physical Activity, Exercise: Health:

  Peacefulness: Accomplishments:

  Happiness: Self-Esteem:

_____

- General Comments, Reactions and any To-Do List:

Chapter 3

Pure Distilled Water for Whole Body Health

Pure distilled water is our choice for health!

You get it from the natural juices of vegetables, fruits and other foods, or from the water of high purity obtained by steam distillation which is the best method. Another effective method combines de-ionization and purification.

The body is constantly working for you, breaking down old bone and tissue cells and replacing them with new ones. As the body casts off old minerals and other products of broken-down cells it must obtain new supplies of essential elements for new cells. Scientists are beginning to understand that various kinds of dental problems, many types of arthritis and some forms of hardening of the arteries are due to imbalances in the body's levels of calcium, phosphorus and magnesium. Disorders can also be caused by imbalances in the ratios of various minerals to each other.

43

Each healthy body requires proper balance within itself of all nutritive elements. It is just as bad to have too much of one item as it is to have too little of another one. It takes appropriate levels of phosphorus and magnesium to keep calcium in solution so it can be formed into new bone and teeth. Yet, there must not be too much of those nor too little calcium in the diet, or old bone will be taken away, but then new bone will not be formed.

The problem of Pharmaceuticals in our drinking water has been an ongoing health issue for decades (www.fda.gov). Polyfluoroalkyl and Perfluoroalkyl (PFASs) exceed federally recommended safety levels in public drinking water supplies. The Agency for Toxic Substances and Disease Registry, say some studies have suggested PFASs are associated with developmental health problems in children, decreased fertility and an increased cancer risk.

Be Safe – Drink Purified Water!

Pure water is vitally important in following *The Bragg Healthy Lifestyle*. Water is the key to all body functions including: circulation, digestion, assimilation, elimination, heart, energy, bones and joints, muscles, nerves, glands and senses. The right kind of water is one of your best natural protections against all kinds of diseases and infections. It is a vital factor in all body fluids, tissues, cells, lymph nodes, blood and all glandular secretions. Water holds all nutritive factors in solution, as well as toxins and body wastes, and acts as the main transportation medium throughout the body, for both nutrition and cleansing purposes (page 50).

Since your body is 75% water, and the blood (plasma) and lymphatic system is over 90% water, it is essential for your health that you drink only pure water not saturated with contaminants, inorganic minerals and toxins. This pure water will transport vital nutrients to cells and waste from cells more efficiently. This allows the body to function correctly and stay healthier!

44

ORGANIC MINERALS: Your minerals must come from an organic source, from something living or that has lived. Humans do not have the same chemistry as plants. Only the living plant has the ability to extract inorganic minerals from the earth and convert them to organic minerals for your body to absorb and utilize them.

INORGANIC MINERALS: The inorganic minerals and toxic chemicals in water can create these problems:

- *Clogs the arteries and small capillaries that are needed to feed and nourish your brain with oxygenated blood; the result is loss of memory and gradual senility and strokes.*
- *Hardens the liver.*
- *Causes kidney stones and gallstones.*
- *Causes arthritis, bone spurs and painful calcified formations in the joints.*

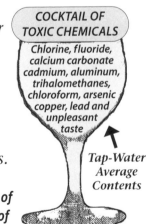

COCKTAIL OF TOXIC CHEMICALS

Chlorine, fluoride, calcium carbonate cadmium, aluminum, trihalomethanes, chloroform, arsenic copper, lead and unpleasant taste

Tap-Water Average Contents

Distilled water plays a vital part in the treatment of illness, arthritis, etc. – Dr. Allen E. Banik, author of "Your Water and Your Health" & "The Choice is Clear"

Water is the Key to All Body Functions!
This is why 8-10 glasses distilled water daily is important

- Heart
- Circulation
- Digestion
- Bones & Joints

- Muscles
- Metabolism
- Assimilation
- Elimination

- Glands
- Sex
- Energy
- Nerves

Pure Distilled Water for Whole Body Health

People who drink sufficient amounts of the right kinds of liquids (distilled water, fresh fruits and veggies and their juices) have better functioning and circulation overall, which is most important to Super Health and Long Life.

You have 15 billion powerful brain cells and the brain is 75% water. We strongly believe the right kind of water in sufficient amounts helps improve your mind and brain power and makes you think better and more accurately!

Remember that the whole body – heart, nerves and colon need the correct amount of pure distilled water to function properly. A simple way to help yourself to better health – drink 8 glasses of distilled water daily!

While we believe that distilled water is optimal, there are excellent water purifiers available, as well as reputable pure water companies, that produce clean, chemical-free and residue-free water. We strongly encourage you to choose a pure water alternative to tap water! You can even buy pure, filtered water at your local health food store if you do not have a water purifier in your home.

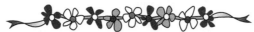

For health's sake it's important to use only purified water.
It's a supreme internal body-cleansing agent.
– Dr. Charles McFerrin, "Nature's Path"

There are thousands of case histories of people who have overcome health problems when they began drinking distilled water.
– Dr. Clifford C. Dennison Ed.D., author "Why I Drink Distilled Water"

The power of pure water is the vital chemistry of all life!

20 FACTS ABOUT DISTILLED WATER

You should know that Distilled Water . . .

- is water that's been turned into vapor so its impurities are left behind. Upon condensing, it becomes pure distilled water.

- is the only type of water which meets the definition of water: hydrogen + oxygen.

- is a perfectly natural healthy water.

- is also odorless, colorless and tasteless.

- is free of virtually all inorganic minerals, including salt.

- is the only natural solvent that can be taken into the body without damage to the tissues.

- acts as a solvent in the body by dissolving nutrients so they can be assimilated and taken into every cell.

- dissolves the cell wastes so the toxins can be removed.

- dissolves inorganic mineral substances lodged in the tissues of the body so that such substances can be eliminated in the process of purifying the body.

- does not leach out organic body minerals but collects and removes the toxic inorganic minerals which have been rejected by the cells and are therefore nothing more than harmful debris obstructing the normal functions of the body.

- is most ideal and beneficial water for all humans and animals.

- leaves no residue of any kind when it enters the body.

- is the most perfect water for the healthy functioning of those great miracle sieves, the kidneys.

- is the perfect liquid for the blood.

- is the ideal liquid for efficient functioning of the lungs, stomach, liver and all other vital organs.

- is universally accepted as the standard for biomedical applications and for drinking water purity.

- is so pure that drug prescriptions are formulated with it.

- is fresh, clean and pleasing to the palate.

- makes foods and drinks prepared with it taste noticeably better. The flavor is subtle enough not to interfere with the food it is mixed with.

- Remember – Distilled Water is the healthiest water and the greatest natural water on earth!

Ten Common Sense Reasons Why We Drink Pure, Distilled Water!

- There are over 80,000 toxic chemicals on the market today . . . and 500 are being added yearly! Regardless of where you live, in the city or on the farm, some of these chemicals are getting into your drinking water.

- No one on the face of the earth today knows what effect these chemicals could have upon the human body as they blend into thousands of different combinations. It is like making a mixture of colors; one drop could change the color.

- The equipment hasn't been designed to detect some of these chemicals and may not be for many years to come.

- The body is made up of 75% water (shown on page 50). Therefore, don't you think you should be particular about the type of water you drink to maintain the health of your miracle body?

- Navy Officers / Sailors have been drinking distilled water for years!

- Distilled water is chemical and mineral free. Distillation removes all the chemicals and impurities from water that are possible to remove. If distillation doesn't remove them, there is no known method that will.

- The body does need minerals . . . but it is not necessary that they come from water. There is not one mineral in water which cannot be found more abundantly in food! Water is the most unreliable source of minerals because it varies from one area to another. The food we eat – not the water we drink – is the best source of organic minerals!

- Distilled water is used for intravenous feeding, inhalation therapy, prescriptions, baby formulas and kidney dialysis. Therefore, doesn't it make common sense that it is good for everyone?

- Thousands of water distillers have been sold throughout the United States and around the world to individuals, families, dentists, doctors, hospitals, nursing homes and government agencies. These and other informed, alert consumers are helping protect their health by using only pure, distilled water. Be health wise – do the same.

- With all of the toxic chemicals, pollutants and other impurities in our water, it only makes good common sense you should clean up the water you drink Mother Nature's wise, inexpensive way through distillation!

Please Don't Drink Water Treated By Water Softeners!

Water softeners are being used in millions of homes because hard water is not ideal for washing your hair, clothes, dishes, etc. If you wash your hair in soft water you will discover how soft it is. *But please do not drink the water out of water softeners!* It is not healthy for you to drink and cook your food with because of its salt and chemical content. It contains suspended inorganic minerals and salts that produce more suds ideal for washing clothes and dishes; but this chemically softened water is harmful to your body.

Use distilled water for drinking and cooking to ensure a longer life and health for you and your family! You will find complete, documented reports on the web of the health hazards of softened water and reasons for drinking only pure distilled water in our book, *Water – The Shocking Truth!* (See back pages for Bragg Book list.)

Keep Toxic Fluoride Out of Your Water!

Most of the water Americans drink has fluoride in it, including tap and bottled water and canned drinks and foods! The ADA (American Dental Association) is insisting that the FDA (Food and Drug Association) mandate the addition of toxic fluoride to all bottled waters! Millions of innocent people have been brainwashed by the aluminum companies to erroneously believe adding sodium fluoride (their waste by-product) to drinking water will reduce tooth decay in our children. Millions of Americans drink a daily dose of sodium fluoride in their water without even knowing it.

To Maximize Body Effectiveness, Drink Water . . .

- in the morning to help activate internal organs.
- before taking a bath/shower to help lower blood pressure.
- two to three hours before bedtime, helps to avoid stroke or heart attack.
- with apple cider vinegar 30 minutes before meals, to help improve digestion, gerd and glucose levels. – Gabriel Cousens, M.D.

Distilled water plays a vital part in the treatment of illness, arthritis, etc. – Dr. Allen E. Banik, author "The Choice is Clear"

Fluorine is a Deadly Poison!

Sodium fluorine, a chemical "cousin" of sodium fluoride, is used as a rat and roach killer and a deadly pesticide! Yet this deadly sodium fluoride, injected almost by government edict into drinking water in the proportion of 1.2 parts per million (PPM), has been declared by the U.S. Public Health Service to be *safe for all*

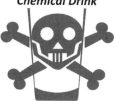

Caution: Toxic Water Chemical Drink

human consumption. Every chemist knows that such absolute safety is not only false but is also truly unattainable and a total illusion!

Studies Show Fluoride Causes Cancer and Many Other Health Problems

- Studies show that fluoridation is causing an increase in bone cancer and deaths among males under 20.

- The growing increase in osteosarcoma is attributable to an increase in toxic fluoride.

- It is causing an increase in oral (mouth) cancer. Don't use fluoride toothpaste or allow your dentist to do fluoride treatments or use fluoride polishing paste!

- Fluoride has been linked to many health problems:
  - bone and oral cancers in humans (even in animals).
  - an ability to inhibit the DNA repair enzyme system.
  - accelerates tumor growth and inhibits immune system.
  - causes genetic damage in cell lines and induces melanotic tumors, fibrosarcomas, and the like.
  - other tumors/cancers strongly indicate fluoride has generalized effect of increasing them overall.

- According to study estimates, thousands of people in the United States die of cancer each year due to fluoridation of their public drinking water.

CHECK FOLLOWING WEBSITES FOR FLUORIDE UPDATES:

- www.FluorideAlert.org • fluoride.mercola.com
- www.slweb.org/bibliography.html
- www.DoctorYourself.com/carton.html

Fluoride is a waste by-product of the fertilizer and aluminum industry and it's also a Part II Poison under the UK Poisons Act 1972.

THE 75% WATERY HUMAN

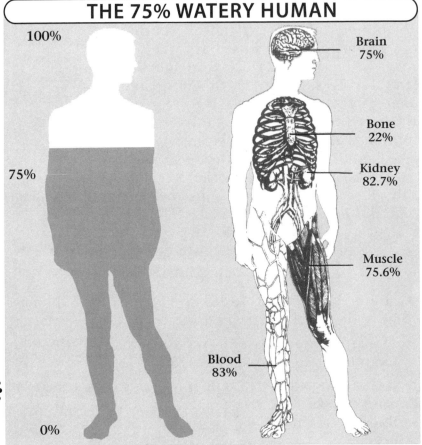

100%

75%

0%

Brain
75%

Bone
22%

Kidney
82.7%

Muscle
75.6%

Blood
83%

The amount of water in human body, averaging 75%, varies considerably even from one part of the body to another area as shown here. A lean man may hold 75% of his weight in body water, while a woman – because of her larger proportion of adipose tissues – may be only 52% water. The lowering of the water content in the blood is what triggers the hypothalamus, the brain's vital thirst center, to send out its familiar urgent demand for a drink of water! Please obey and drink ample amounts (8 glasses) of purified, distilled water daily. By the time you feel thirsty, you're already dehydrated. – American Running & Fitness Association

WATER PERCENTAGE IN VARIOUS BODY PARTS:

Teeth	10%	Spleen	75.5%
Bones	22%	Lungs	80%
Cartilage	55%	Blood	83%
Red blood corpuscles	68.7%	Bile	86%
Liver	71.5%	Plasma	90%
Brain	75%	Lymph	94%
Muscle tissue	75%	Saliva	95.5%

This chart shows why 8-10 glasses of pure water daily is so important.

Chapter 4

The "Gravity" of the Situation

Excess weight overloads your body, spine and feet

Why should emphasis be placed upon such a simple thing as the pull of gravity? This is very easy to explain. In youth, as long as your muscles were strong enough, they held your skeleton in proper balance with its many points and sections free from strain or discomfort. As your body ages, your muscles start to lose the battle with gravity, especially if you are prematurely ageing or heavier than you should be, or a forced rest has weakened your muscles just enough to cause an uncomfortable state of body imbalance.

When you consider that 1,300 pounds of pull are exerted on your spine and sacroiliac joints simply to maintain an erect posture, and that practically the entire weight of your vital organs is borne by the spine, you can understand why an excess burden of fat usually results in chronic backache and tired feet.

51

Being overweight exacts many other health penalties too! It over-burdens the heart with fatty tissue and forces the heart to strain with over-work in pumping blood through the additional miles of blood vessels. Often high blood pressure develops from obesity, as well as adult-onset diabetes! Diabetes can cause problems with your feet, see pages 179-183. Fat deposits impede the functioning of vital organs, such as the heart, lungs, kidneys and pancreas.

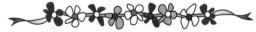

Healthy organic foods have a wonderful abundance of potential life energy.

To our minds the greatest mistake a person can make is to remain ignorant when he is surrounded everyday of his life, with the knowledge he needs to grow and be healthy, happy and successful. It's all there – you need only observe, read, learn and then apply the wisdom. – Paul C. Bragg, N.D., Ph.D.

What is "Normal Weight?"

There are numerous charts, tables and statistics on the subject of normal weight for your age, height, etc. These are based on averages. However, there is no such thing as an average person. You may use such statistics as a general guide, but they should not be applied arbitrarily to determine your exact healthiest weight.

If you give your body the proper, healthy diet and ample exercise, you will naturally attain and maintain your best personal weight! To weigh a certain number of pounds does not necessarily indicate your proper measurement of waist, hips, etc. If you are firm and healthy – it doesn't matter whether you weigh more or less than the chart average for your years and height. The important thing is to find your own best weight as the result of proper care you give your body. If your body is healthy, trim and fit, then your weight is normal for you.

Your Waistline is Your Life-line, Youth-line, Date-line and Health-line

When you have a "spare tire" you are flirting with premature old age! Carrying excess belly fat impairs lung function (*reuters.com*). Abdominal obesity is defined as having a waistline of greater than 35" for women and 40" for men. French Researchers think belly fat may impair the way the diaphragm and chest function. Surplus weight in the belly lessens physical activity and often mental activity, too. Don't be satisfied thinking that a naturally fatty surplus comes with advancing years! Beware if you make this mistake, for old age will arrive sooner coupled with serious illness and premature death.

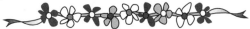

Eating high-quality, organic, bio-dynamic, locally-grown food will naturally increase your bone density and decrease your risk of developing osteoporosis. Along with your foods, your omega-3 fat content also has a major role in building healthy bone. I recommend krill oil, as I believe it's a superior source of omega-3s. – Dr. Mercola • www.mercola.com

It's strange that some men will drink and eat anything put before them, but will check very carefully the oil they put in their car.

"Visceral Fat" Linked to Heart Disease, Diabetes, Stroke & Other Chronic Diseases*

Your body has two types of fat: visceral and subcutaneous. Subcutaneous fat is found just under your skin and causes dimpling and cellulite. Visceral fat shows up in your abdomen and surrounds your vital organs including your liver, heart and muscles. Visceral fat spells trouble for your health. It drives up your risk for diabetes, heart disease, stroke, and even dementia.

If you are eating a diet that is high in white sugar and refined grains (see page 26-29) – this is the same type of diet that will also increase inflammation in your body, as the sugar gets metabolized in fat cells, fat releases surges in *leptin*. Over time, if your body is exposed to too much leptin, it will become resistant to the leptin (just as your body can become resistant to insulin).

When you become *leptin-resistant*, your body can no longer hear the messages telling it to stop eating and burn fat – so it remains hungry and stores more fat. Leptin-resistance also causes an increase in visceral fat, sending you on a vicious cycle of hunger, fat storage and an increased risk of heart disease, diabetes and more.

53

How You Can Stop "Visceral Fat"

Avoid eating pro-inflammatory foods such as white sugar, soda, alcohol, refined grains and trans fats (see list of "Foods to Avoid" page 38). Foods that will reduce inflammation are fruits and vegetables, omega-3 fats like fish oil and certain spices like ginger (see page 56).

Exercise is critical! Exercise is one of the best weapons to fight visceral fat – it drastically reduces visceral fat and lowers inflammation. One study found that volunteers who did not exercise had an 8.6% increase in visceral fat after 8 months, while those who exercised the most lost over 8% of their visceral fat during that time.

So whether you are thin or carrying excess belly fat, going on a healthy nutrition plan and exercise program will do wonders for your future health and longevity.

***Excerpt From Dr. Mercola article • www.mercola.com**

Keeping Trim & Fit Good For Your Self-Esteem!

Self-esteem is as necessary to the spirit as healthful food is to the body. If you want to be efficient, eternally youthful, enthusiastic, full of fire and fervor of life, keep trim and fit and protect your self-esteem! Build your body as an artist paints a picture or a sculptor molds a statue. Make your body an expression of the best there is within you! Let it reflect your soul and true self. Give thanks, as soon excess fat will find no lodging on your frame and in your flesh!

Be Your Body's Health Captain

In our years as authors, nutritionists and physical life-coaches, we have helped millions of men and women attain and maintain healthy, normal weight by natural methods! We know of no other sure way to accomplish lifelong weight control than by living a healthy lifestyle and establishing a regular regimen of diet and exercise that keeps your metabolism in proper balance. Metabolism is the intricate process by which your body converts food to energy. When you take in more fuel (food) than you burn up in energy (activities), the excess is stored as fat in the less used body areas!

Maintain Healthy Natural Diet for Health

A natural foods diet is the best way to maintain a normal weight and good health. In Mother Nature's design for living, she has provided perfectly balanced nutrition for every living thing in both the plant and animal kingdoms.

However, in attempting to redesign this pattern for their own convenience, humans have upset this balance, and are paying the penalty in loss of health. Modern civilization has opted for pre-packaged convenience over natural foods. The resulting need for mass transportation, storage and distribution of food has transformed the average diet into an artificial one, made up primarily of devitalized, processed, additive-ridden dead fast foods, which might satisfy hunger, but not the body's health demands. In the last

60 years, the American diet has deteriorated such that millions of children and adults walk around obese and malnourished, with low energy and weak, slumped spines. In a desperate effort to get a lift, millions resort to drugs; from slow killers (cola drinks, caffeine, alcohol and nicotine) to those that are more speedily fatal.

Is it possible to live on a natural diet in this polluted world? Yes, it is! It requires some dedicated, strong effort and wise discrimination, but the rewards are great. Isn't it worth your effort to exchange the misery of an unhealthy life for the joy of a vital, glowing, healthy life?

"Good Earth" Founder Thanks Bragg Books

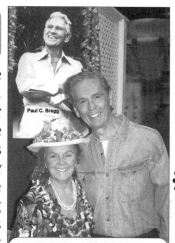

Bill Galt, founder of The Good Earth Restaurant chain, charged himself with super health and changed his entire life after reading Bragg books *Miracle of Fasting* and *The Bragg Healthy Lifestyle*. His entire family followed The Bragg Healthy Lifestyle. Their friends and associates wanted to know what was the cause of the miraculous changes they saw in

Patricia with Bill Galt and Paul Bragg's Picture

55

the Galts! Their friends wanted what they had – super health! Bill and his family started a tiny restaurant that served only lunches. An overnight success, they started serving a full vegetarian menu all day. Soon they expanded and opened a chain of health restaurants, all serving delicious healthy food based on The Bragg Healthy Lifestyle! We were blessed to have a Good Earth Restaurant in Santa Barbara. Many Hollywood Stars often ate there, including Jack LaLanne.

Many people go through their life committing partial suicide.
They destroy their health, youth, talents, energies and creative qualities.
Indeed, to learn how to be good to oneself is often harder than
to learn how to be good to others. – Joshua Liebman, Ph.D.,
American Rabbi, best-selling author "Peace of Mind"

Getting the Body Back into Healthy Balance

Dr. Mark Hyman (*drhyman.com*) and Dr. Mercola (*mercola.com*) recommend the following simple effective ways to achieve balance and reduce your inflammation:

1. Eat Whole Foods: choose unprocessed, unrefined, whole, real foods, such as organic fruits and vegetables, whole grains, legumes, nuts and seeds (see pages 22-24).

2. Have Healthy Fats: getting more omega-3 fats in olive oil, nuts and avocados (see page 24).

3. Eat foods that improve your insulin sensitivity: raw, unfiltered apple cider vinegar (with the *mother*), green tea (decaffeinated), nuts and spices such as ginger, cinnamon and turmeric.

4. Exercise Regularly: regular exercise helps reduce inflammation. It also improves your immune function, strengthens your cardiovascular system, corrects and prevents insulin resistance, and is key for improving your mood and erasing effects of stress! In fact, regular exercise will improve health in virtually ALL areas of your life. Now get busy moving, exercising, and living healthy!

5. Relax your whole body: it lowers inflammation, also practice yoga, meditation and prayer, breathe slowly and deeply, read, take a relaxing hot shower or bath.

6. Avoid Allergens: find out what you're allergic to and stop eating those foods (see Dr. Coca's Pulse Test and the list of "Most Common Food Allergies" page 39).

7. Heal Your Gut: take pro-biotics and drink apple cider vinegar (see recipe page 40). Both help digestion and improve the balance of healthy bacteria in your gut, which helps to reduce body inflammation.

8. Supplements: take a multi-vitamin/multi-mineral supplement, fish oil and vitamin D3, all help reduce body inflammation.

Taking steps to reduce inflammation and balance your immune system address the core system of the body – your precious miracle blood! It's the basis of healthy living.

Humor is healthy – it improves blood circulation, boosts immune system, and helps relieve stress. – Dr. Joel Goodman, "Laffirmations"

Chapter 5

Walking – The King of Exercise

Keep your entire body fit and healthy!

About 2,400 years ago, Hippocrates said, "Walking is man's best medicine." More recently, the consensus of those at the National Institutes of Health was that walking is the most efficient form of exercise and the only one you can wisely follow safely all the years of your life.

There is nothing as pleasurable as walking. When taking a walk, open your eyes wide and keep your mind receptive to what is around you: see new flowers blooming, hear birds singing. To enjoy the various seasons of Mother Nature is so rewarding to watch because each season has its own individual beauty!

If our feet are *killing* us or our backs are *stiff*, all the joys of walking are gone. Many people forego the pleasure of walking because their feet and back cry out in pain with every step.

Walking is one of the best overall exercises to keep your feet, back and entire body happy, fit and healthy! It is the king of exercises and can be enjoyed alone or with a group of people. It is something everyone at all ages can participate in: children, students, working people, retired persons and seniors. There is always a way to incorporate walking into your lifestyle; walking to school, the store, to work, etc. Park a little distance away from where you are going and walk the rest of the way.

Walking utilizes our 260 bones, 640 muscles and 70,000 miles of circulatory channels. Every part of the body benefits from walking! Barring disabling injuries or conditions, walking comes as naturally to us as breathing. A regular walking program will increase lung capacity and actually improve your breathing patterns while improving your circulation and health!

The Medical Journal "Circulation" reports that people who don't make efforts to exercise regularly face the same dangerous risk of heart disease as people who smoke a pack of cigarettes daily.

Benefits of Walking are Abundant

The muscles of the feet, calves, thighs, buttocks, back and abdomen all work when you walk. The oxygen your body needs to function properly is distributed more effectively. The heart works harder, sending blood coursing through your veins to improve your entire circulation. Even low or moderate-intensity walking can offer many important cardiovascular benefits, according to medical researchers. Regular walking: three to four times a week for 30 to 60 minutes, depending on intensity, can help normalize cholesterol, blood pressure, elimination and also fights osteoporosis.

Walking also reduces anxiety and tension and aids in weight loss. There are 3,500 calories in a pound of fat. If an overweight person walks just 20 minutes a day and does not change their eating habits, they can start losing weight.

Other benefits include the strengthening and toning of muscles, weight control and ridding the body of toxins through perspiration. A regular exercise program such as walking also has a tremendously positive effect on mental attitude. Just the act of getting out and doing something physical is, in itself, a mood elevator. The increase of blood circulation in the brain lifts the spirits, calms you down and makes you feel more self-confident. There are also chemical reactions caused by brisk walking that increase the level of endorphins, which are vital chemicals in the body that make us feel good!

Walking is an exercise that needs no gym, natural medicine that requires no prescription, weight control without a diet, a cosmetic not sold in a drugstore. It is the tranquilizer without a pill, the therapy without a psychoanalyst, the fountain of youth that is no legend. A walk is a healthy mini-vacation that does not cost a cent. So, it's easy to see that there is nothing to lose and everything to gain by investing in a good pair of walking shoes and going for a healthy fun walk.

Nothing is more important as you age than staying physically active and eating a healthy diet with lots of fresh, organic fruits and vegetables.
– Jane Fonda • www.JaneFonda.com

The Bragg Philosophy of Walking

Walk naturally with head high, chest up, feeling physically elated. Carry yourself proudly, straight, erect and with an easy action of swinging arms. Go at your own stride and with your spirit free. If the world of Mother Nature fails to interest you, turn to the inner world of the spirit. As you walk, your body ceases to matter and you become as near to being a poet as ever you will be, each step bringing you inspiration.

Enjoy Your Walk – Leisure or Brisk

There are two different kinds of walks you can take, the leisurely stroll and the brisk, disciplined walk designed for maximum isotonic (heart and circulatory) benefit. If you haven't been involved in an exercise program for a while, walking is the perfect way to get back into the exercise habit. It helps condition you for other activities such as aerobics, jogging or competitive sports like tennis, cycling and swimming and skiing.

As with any new activity undertaken, it's important to start slowly and to know your limits. If you are over 35 or have been inactive because of illness, etc, ask your health professional to give you a treadmill stress test. This helps determine whether your heart can tolerate continuous high-speed walking or leisurely walking.

An old Spanish proverb says, "Walk 'til the blood appears in the cheeks, but not the sweat on the brow," and is good wise advice for novice walkers. Here are some guidelines on proper walking techniques. What you don't want to do is to walk slumped over with toes pointed outward, arms flailing and feet landing flatfooted. Your head and back should be erect and shoulders relaxed with arms swinging. The buttocks should be tucked in slightly, even when walking. The toes should be pointed straight ahead when walking and remember your big toes are your foot captains! When walking your eyes should be looking at least 4 yards ahead. Walking with straight posture, *and lifting up your chest*, gives the walker a higher center of gravity and a longer stride.

If you don't use it, you lose it – it's also true for the mind, body and spirit.

The arms should swing naturally in an arc about the shoulder. For a faster walking style, bend the arms 90° at the elbows so the arms can match the quicker leg movements. *(Some walkers like to use hand weights.)* Exhale and inhale breathing deeply and rhythmically, counting one breath for each one, two, or more steps. Soon, this super breathing style becomes second nature. Do read the *Bragg Super Power Breathing* book for more breathing exercises (see back pages for booklist).

When smooth striding, the heel should land first. Strive to eliminate any up-and-down or side-to-side movements and concentrate on smooth fluid forward movements for a flowing comfortable walking gait.

On your first four days out, simply walk what is comfortable for you. One sports expert recommends beginning with 15-25 minutes of walking three times a week. (Don't forget that you also have to walk back unless you arrange for a ride at the other end, which is a little self-defeating if done beyond the first week.) On the fifth day, increase your distance by 25%. Five days later, increase the new distance by another 25% and so on.

Start out with a walking pace that doesn't create a strain. Distance is more important than speed. It's advisable to wait until you've been walking regularly for at least a month before you pick up the pace, and then only speed up to a pace that is comfortable for you. The U.S. Army recommends a pace of 3 miles per hour. This is based on the length of stride and standard height of the average American male. Most women walkers, despite a shorter average height, can handle this pace without strain, once they've reached a level of good overall fitness and health conditioning.

The important thing, however, is to find a stride speed that feels good to you! If you find, using a pedometer, that you're walking less than 3 mph but feel you're getting a good workout without overexerting yourself, then this is the pace you should maintain. At the 3 mph rate, one mile should take you about 20 minutes – a pleasant time that passes quickly once you get into the spirit of the walk and enjoy the scenery and quietness.

Walking Energizes and Refreshes

Make your walking a priority and stick with it. If you have a hard time getting yourself going, try the buddy system. Make arrangements with a family member, friend or neighbor to call each other on a rotating basis. Having someone to encourage and support your efforts definitely helps. It also gives you the responsibility of helping them. Besides, both of you will benefit from having someone to talk to about how great your life is becoming on the walk to make those miles slip away!

Another way to keep your interest level high is to vary the route you take. This can be done on a daily, weekly or strictly random basis. Make a deal with yourself to notice 10 new sights on your walk each day. This will not be difficult. Plan to make each walk an exciting adventure! Make the most of your walking! Enjoy the tranquility that comes with appreciating Mother Nature's wonders. As you walk, pray, meditate or sing, *Health, Strength, Youth, Vitality, Joy, Peace* and *Fulfillment* for *Eternity!* Sing or say it silently, shout it out or make up a song to keep time with your stride. Just make sure the message is positive and reinforcing! Make it part of your walking program. It will reward you in many ways beyond happy feet and a healthy body!

When You Are Ready for Jogging - Prepare

Once you have hit 5 to 6 miles of walking at a steady pace, you may feel inclined to start jogging. By this time your muscles, lungs, heart and mind will have become conditioned for a more strenuous workout. But, again, be sure to check with your doctor if you have any concerns about overloading your body and its systems.

Work into jogging gradually. Walk at maximum speed for five minutes and then jog for 60 seconds at a slow pace. Then walk again, followed by another 60 second jog. Alternate jogging and walking about five times. Do this for a week and then gradually increase your jogging.

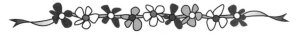

Just as the body flourishes on a healthy diet, our joy flourishes with mother nature's beauty. – Thomas Kinkade • www.ThomasKinkade.com

As soon as you feel confident that you're not putting undue stress on your heart, feet, back or leg muscles, add another 10 to 20 seconds and decrease your walking time by the same amount. Generally, it is advised by sports experts that you wait one to two weeks between these changes.

Within a few months, you should be able to do light jogging non-stop for 20 to 30 minutes and you may also want to add more speed to your workout. But remember, your body is the best judge of your capabilities! Trust it and be aware of any signs that may be an indication that you are overdoing it. A few "trouble signals" to be aware of are extreme short-windedness, dizziness, sharp pains in any muscles, joints or bones, cramps, chest pain or a sudden feeling of fatigue.

Take Precautions to Avoid Injuries

If you experience any of the aforementioned "trouble signals," stop jogging immediately and rest or resume walking at a reduced pace. Sometimes the symptom is a temporary warning that you are creating stress on certain body areas. By slowing down, many aches, pains and reactions will simply disappear. However, if any of the symptoms persist or become uncomfortable, it's wise to see your doctor before starting to jog again.

You would not consider entering a professional auto race without having a finely tuned, specially designed car under you to insure peak performance. The same principle applies to jogging. You need those finely tuned, specially designed shoes to maximize your efforts and reduce the possibility of any breakdown of your precious body's equipment.

I have the wisdom of my years and the youthfulness of
The Bragg Healthy Lifestyle and I never act or feel
my calendar years! I feel ageless! Then why shouldn't you?
Start living this Bragg Healthy Way today!
– Patricia Bragg, Health Crusader

The American diet is overloaded with too much food and the harmful fats that raise blood cholesterol levels that can cause fatal heart disease!

The Optimum Stretch

You can easily incur sprains and pulled muscles or tendonitis by hitting your stride without first warming up. A pre-jog walk will help loosen the body and prepare you for greater exertion. However, the best and most effective warm-up is simple, slow stretching. It's the safest way to elongate the muscles and increase flexibility.

Stretching expert Bob Anderson, a Bragg follower for years, recommends stretching for 8 to 10 minutes before and after jogging. He also suggests that you feel free to take short stretching breaks at any time during your jog, walk or run when you experience soreness or tension. For more information see Anderson's website and book: *www.stretching.com*

A good stretch should be done smoothly and slowly, without any jerking or bouncing motions. Stretch to the point where you feel a slight tension on the muscles and hold for 10 seconds. The longer you hold the stretch, the less tension you should feel. Never *push* the stretch or put prolonged tension on the muscles.

Return to your starting position, relax for a few seconds and then stretch again, moving into the stretch a bit further so you experience slight tension. Hold for 10 seconds. If the tension does not diminish, ease off to a more comfortable position. Stretching should never be a strain! If you find that at first you can not fully reach a position or can only stay in the position for a short time, do not worry. You will soon notice an increase in flexibility by stretching regularly.

It is not necessary to limit your stretching to before and after a workout. In fact, it is a method of relaxation that can be incorporated into your daily life: at work, in the morning to limber up, after a long meeting or anytime you feel like it! Don't forget to exercise and stretch toes and feet to keep them strong and flexible.

63

"If I had to pick one thing . . . that came closest to the fountain of youth, it would be exercise." Exercising just 15 minutes a day helps maintain healthy blood vessels for good circulation in the body and brain.
– James Fries, M.D., expert on ageing at Stanford University in California

Healthy Walking Rejuvenates the Body

Walking is actually like a series of falls aborted by muscular force. When you realize this, you can better understand why it is so important to the health of your spine and feet to walk correctly. When you *walk tall,* with a full-length lifted-up spine, the shock absorbers of your spinal column (*cartilage plates and discs*) have room to function well. Your spine will act as a spring, protecting the spinal cord and the brain from jolts of each step.

Continued pavement pounding takes its toll on spinal resiliency by subjecting your shock absorbers to undue stress. Shoes with low rubber heels and flexible rubber soles, help to cushion the shock! Your feet are springy levers that carry the weight of your body forward with each step. Although they need protection from hard pavement, they must not be confined or cramped; they need freedom of action in well-fitted shoes.

If you have pain or discomfort in walking, the three key points to check are your feet, shoes and spine. The Spine Motion Exercises, the Foot Program and stretching exercises in this book will help greatly to make walking the buoyant, joyous exercise it is naturally supposed to be. You should gracefully swing along as though your legs begin in the middle of your torso, using your back, side and abdominal muscles as well as thigh, leg and foot muscles. Let arms swing rhythmically from your shoulders. Hold head tall, and walk proud! **Walking as Nature intended is the energizing *King of Exercise* that helps rejuvenate the entire body!**

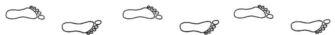

I never suspected that I would have to learn how to live – that there were specific disciplines and ways of seeing the world that I had to master before I could awaken to a simple, healthy, happy, uncomplicated life.
– Dan Millman - A Bragg fan since Stanford University coaching days.

I used to say, "I sure hope things will change." Then, I learned that the only way things are going to change for me is when I change!
– Jim Rohn

To desire to be healthy is part of being healthy. – Seneca

Chapter 6

The Importance of Good Posture

Proper posture is continuous exercise

Before we go into the special Spine Motion Exercises and Foot Program, we must establish the basic exercise, which should be so thoroughly programmed into your nervous system that you practice it all the time: *standing, sitting, walking, lying down.* This continuous exercise is habit of proper posture. It begins in infancy and continues throughout life!

Posture means the position we hold our bodies. Proper posture is the balanced alignment of the body. When standing erect, an imaginary plumb line representing the center of gravity should fall in alignment with the top center of the skull through the center of the ear, and through the centers of the joints at the shoulder, to the rest of the body; shoulders straight; chest up and not in an exaggerated stance; keep abdomen firm and lift chest up off of waist. In this position, the spine holds its natural, gentle curves, and the weight of the body is supported by the hips and feet, slightly apart, with stress on the heels.

To sum it up, *Stand tall!* To get that tall feeling, imagine that a powerful giant is holding you by the hair and almost lifting you off the ground! You should not only *stand tall, you must also sit tall and walk tall and sleep tall!* If you have been slouching or slumping, as most people do, you will probably find that this erect posture is uncomfortable at first, because your muscles and ligaments have become too slack or too tense from being held in the wrong positions and not properly exercised.

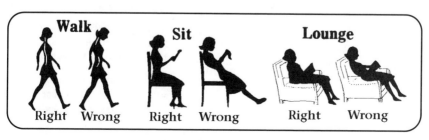

Walk		Sit		Lounge	
Right	Wrong	Right	Wrong	Right	Wrong

Let Your Mirror Be Your Personal Judge

Check your own posture and your symptoms (below and page 67). Do you notice a deep aching and soreness along your spine due to stretched ligaments? Are your back and shoulder areas achy and tired? Is your backache due basically to weak muscles? If it is, it's about time you did something sensible to relieve it, like strengthening all those weak muscles by proper exercise and posture.

To find out literally *the true shape you're in,* stand in front of a full-length mirror and critically view yourself as you would a stranger. Examine your front. Using the reflection from a hand mirror, examine your sides and then your back. Wear a swimsuit, or nothing at all! Let your mirror mercilessly reveal shocking truths.

Does your head stick forward? Do your shoulders slump? Is one shoulder or hip higher than the other? Is your upper back round? Do you have a pot belly? Are you swayback? Does your spine curve to one side?

Analyze your posture defects (see below and next page) and list by date on a chart. Keep weekly record of your progress toward perfect posture, reexamining yourself in the mirror each week as you carry out this Back and Foot Fitness Program. Faithfully follow the instructions in this book and soon you will be highly gratified by the results, in both health and a more youthful appearance and well-being!

Posture Silhouettes: Which one are you?

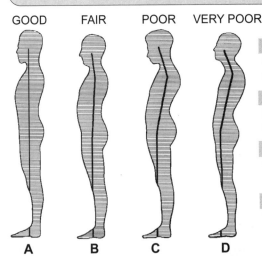

GOOD   FAIR   POOR   VERY POOR

A Good: Head, trunk and thigh in a straight line; chest high and forward; abdomen flat; back curves normally.

B Fair: Head too forward; abdomen too prominent; exaggerated curve in upper back; slightly hollow lower back.

C Poor: Relaxed posture; head too forward; abdomen relaxed; shoulder blades prominent; hollow lower back.

D Very Poor: Head too far forward; very exaggerated curve in upper back; abdomen relaxed; chest flat-sloping.

A   B   C   D

WHERE DO YOU STAND?

POSTURE CHART

	PERFECT	FAIR	POOR
HEAD			
SHOULDERS			
SPINE			
HIPS			
ANKLES			
NECK			
UPPER BACK			
TRUNK			
ABDOMEN			
LOWER BACK			

A healthy, flexible, aligned spine goes a long way in helping you to stay youthful for a long, active, healthy, fulfilled life!

Remember – Your posture can make or break your looks and health!

Good Posture Habits Important For Health

To maintain oneself in a healthy state involves many factors: the right natural food, rest, exercise, sleep, fasting, control of emotions and mind and good posture. If a body is properly nourished and cared for, good posture is not a problem. When the body lacks the essentials, poor posture is often the result. Once poor habits have been established, one must faithfully each day practice corrective exercises and good posture habits!

Paul C. Bragg repeatedly stated, to maintain good health the body must be exercised properly (walking, jogging, biking, swimming, deep breathing, stretching, calisthenics, and good posture) and nourished wisely (healthy natural foods), so as to provide and increase the good life of radiant health, joy and happiness.

Bragg Posture Exercise Brings Miracles
Do This Exercise Daily and Practice Good Posture!

Here's a simple way to check and reset your posture every day. Before a mirror, stand up tall with your feet 10" apart, stretch your spine up. Tighten buttocks, suck in stomach muscles. Move hands up to your lower rib cage, stretch up spine and lift rib cage up. Move hands to upper chest; lift chest up. Move hands to shoulders; lift them up and slightly back. Put right hand under chin and lift chin up. Now line body up straight, nose plumb-line to belly button, and drop hands heavy to sides, swinging them easily back and forth. This normalizes posture naturally and helps you find the posture best for you. Look in the mirror to see if your shoulders are level. You may have to lift one shoulder up a little to equalize and level them. Usually, with practice, they will become naturally level in a week or so, but keep checking them!

By doing this simple posture exercise, miraculous changes will happen! Your body machinery will have more room to operate and your upper body will not compress your vital organs in the chest and abdomen. Bragg Posture Exercise will retrain your frame to sit, stand and walk tall for supreme health, fitness and longevity!

Correct Posture While You Stand, Sit, Walk and Sleep

First you must use your mind to direct your body. We are believers in healthy conscious control of the body. All moves should be first thought-out before they are executed. Most people move their bodies without any conscious direction and this is the reason their bodies, particularly their posture, feet and spine deteriorate and can bring on grave and painful physical problems.

Standing, walking, laying, sitting and getting up from the sitting position must be done correctly to promote correct use of foot, knee and hip joints. The greater majority of people, when they sit in a chair, "flop" into the chair. Or, instead of using their movable body joints, they use the chair arms to get into and out of it. In doing this they are not using the feet, knee or hip joints properly. Years of "flopping" have caused the bones of the feet, knees and hip joints to deteriorate. Not only is damage done to these parts of the body, but the "flopping" into chairs also shocks all 24 movable bones of the spine. This can slowly wear away the discs between the vertebrae and bones of the spine. Soon bones are pressing upon bones, impinging on and damaging nerves that affect many parts of the body adversely.

69

How to Walk Correctly for Health

When walking, one should imagine that the legs are attached to the middle of the chest. This gives long, sweeping, graceful, springy steps, because when one walks correctly with this full swing and spring, one automatically builds energy.

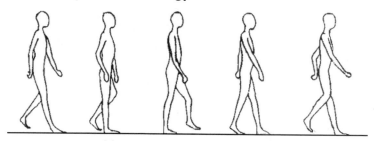

CORRECT WALKING POSTURE:
Always prepare a new base before leaving the old base.

The Art of Healthy Sitting

When in a sitting position, see that the spine is stretched up and you have your back against the chair so that the abdominal cavity is not relaxed, but drawn in some. Have your shoulders back, with your head held high, never jutting forward. Have your arms and hands relaxed in your lap. Never clasp arms (vice-like) around your chest and heart! This is a bad habit that impedes your circulation.

Slouching in a deep chair or sofa, just like slumping over a desk or table, distorts your spine. In different ways, this puts stress and strain in the wrong places (stretching some ligaments and muscles unduly, tensing others to compensate). This can jam some of the vertebrae together, while pulling others out of place.

In sitting as well as standing, the same basic rules of posture apply from the hips upward, to the trunk and head, both supported by the spine and its interconnecting musculoskeletal structure. The base of your spine should be at the rear of the chair seat (which should be flat and straight), and your back against the chair back, which should fit the natural, gentle spine curves. The stomach then should be flat and firm (not relaxed outward), shoulders straight and head high. In other words, *stretch up your spine and sit tall!*

The flat chair seat should be shorter than the thighs, so the edge of the chair does not press against big arteries under the knees. The height from seat to floor should be the length of the legs, with feet resting flat on the floor. Adults who have shorter legs should use a box or footstool. We love rocking chairs – you can get rest by sitting, plus enjoy peaceful rocking exercise!

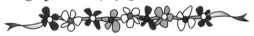

Standing posture is important – stand and walk tall, stretch up your spine so all your middle body machinery is not cramped – your ears, shoulders, hips and knees should be in even balanced line with one another.

Sitting for long periods of time can increase oxidative stress on the body's cells, burden the heart, cause varicose veins, worsen hormone balance, increase the risks for colon cancer and hinder body's vital circulation!

Don't Cross Your Legs – It's Unhealthy

When sitting, please sit correctly! *The* 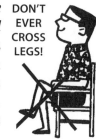 *most disastrous and injurious habit of bad sitting is crossing the legs* for it compresses the popliteal artery in back of knees which can cause a variety of unhealthy problems (blood stagnation in your hips, legs, knees, feet as well as backaches, varicose veins [see below], hemorrhoids, headaches, pain, etc.). Crossing one leg over the other throws the spine out of alignment and can bring on lower back pain and its problems! In women, this unhealthy habit can cause certain disturbances in female organs and, in a man, it may initiate prostate problems.

DON'T EVER CROSS LEGS!

Varicose Veins Can Be Prevented & Reduced

Varicose veins (*Varicosis*) are a result of lifestyle and heredity! While our genetics may determine what we may be susceptible to, lifestyle is an entirely different story. Beyond hereditary predisposition, varicose veins are attributable to poor diet, lack of exercise, circulation and may be helped and prevented by these wise steps:

- **Absolutely do not cross your legs!** Crossing your legs is entirely unnatural; it reduces the blood-flow and constricts veins.

- **Enjoy walking exercises** which promotes circulation.

- **Maintain a healthy diet**, with green leafy vegetables high in vitamin K, such as: kale, Brussel sprouts, spinach, asparagus, and broccoli. A lack of vitamin K is suspected to cause varicose veins.

- **Enjoy fermented foods:** fermented soy products, kimchi, sauerkraut, pickled cucumbers, kefir, yogurt.

- **Avoid constipation** by eating ample fiber and avoid salt, alcohol, and toxins. It's important to drink 8-10 glasses of purified water daily – add raw, organic apple cider vinegar to three of them! After your dinner meal take one psyllium husk capsule daily.

Good posture is a way of doing things with more energy, less stress and fatigue. Without good posture, you cannot really be physically fit.

Stand and Walk Whenever Possible!

Long amounts of sitting are bad for your health. Sitting over 6 hours total per day is shown to put a person at higher risk of dying from cardiovascular disease. Sitting may reduce one's lifespan by years as the more one sits, the less the body wishes to move! Studies show reducing the time spent sitting by only 66 minutes daily, a sedentary person can experience 54% reduction in back and neck pain and can increase their life expectancy by an additional 2 years!

Scientists determined after an hour or more of sitting, the production of enzymes that burn fat in the body declines by about 90%. Extended sitting slows metabolism of glucose and lowers levels of good (HDL) cholesterol in the blood – both being risk factors toward developing heart disease and Type 2 Diabetes.

Some Standing While at Work Can Change and Improve Your Life!

Standing desks offer many health benefits. Standing allows your body to adjust and move – flexing your muscles helps keep your blood circulating. You burn more calories throughout the day (standing burns a third more calories than sitting). This will help you maintain a healthier weight. Standing while working helps fight off the slumps of fatigue that often happen mid-morning or early afternoon. Standing while working helps alleviate back pain and other repetitive stress injuries. When you sit you don't hold your upper body with your muscles, you let the chair hold you. This leads to compression within the chest and abdominal cavities, shoulder slouching and rolling of the spine. These are classic causes for repetitive stress injuries and back pain! Working part-time at a standing desk helps keep your core and back muscles more active and standing tall improves your posture!

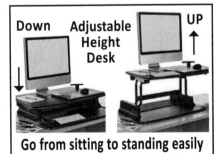

Go from sitting to standing easily with an adjustable stand up desk.

Keep Your Spine Aligned in Bed

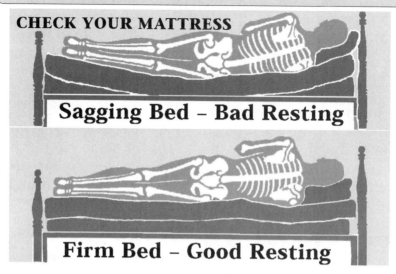

CHECK YOUR MATTRESS

Sagging Bed – Bad Resting

Firm Bed – Good Resting

Your spine must be in proper alignment while you are lying down, whether for a rest, a nap or a good night's sleep. After all, we spend about a third of our lives sleeping! Sleeping on the wrong kind of mattress can throw your spine out of alignment.

A *soft, sagging mattress* fails to give proper support to the heaviest part of the body, the pelvic region and thus causes the spine to curve toward the side on which the person is sleeping. A completely rigid mattress causes curvature in the opposite direction because it does not give sufficiently to accommodate the wider hip and shoulder areas. Neither gives the back or spine the proper kind of support when lying on the back or stomach. Before buying a mattress, lie on it, see how you like it. You do not need box springs; just put your mattress on a wood platform. A memory foam mattress topper can also greatly increase comfort.

Look for a semi-rigid mattress, firm and flat (one with sufficient resilience to allow shoulder and pelvic bones to form their own natural hollows), this helps keep the spinal column in natural alignment. Place a wide bed board between the mattress and box springs to convert most mattresses (except an innerspring mattress) into a semi-rigid mattress.

Good posture helps prevent backaches and related health problems.

The well-known orthopedist Dr. Philip Lewin, in his book *The Back and Its Disorders,* advises us to stand tall, sit tall and adds, laying tall and on your back is the best to align your spine. If on your back, roll a small towel to support the lower back and a pillow under your knees. Sleep with a slanted, cradle pillow that elevates your head. If on your side, put a pillow between your knees. Before you sleep relax all your muscles, go limp, let yourself feel heavy on your bed. Never let one part of your body press on the other as this impedes circulation, keep your arms and legs apart. Neck tension is often due to tensed facial muscles, so think pleasant thoughts that make you feel like smiling.

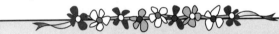

10 Health Benefits of A Good Night's Sleep

- **Improve Your Memory:** During sleep you strengthen memories.

- **Live Longer:** Sleep also affects your quality of life. Too much or too little sleep (8-9 hours optimal) is associated with a shorter lifespan.

- **Curb Inflammation:** Study found C-Reactive Protein was higher in people who got less than 6 hours sleep. Inflammation is linked to heart disease, stroke, diabetes, arthritis and premature ageing.

- **Lower Stress:** Sleep reduces stress levels and people can have better control of their blood pressure, to avoid cardiovascular disease.

- **Improve Grades:** In a study, college students who didn't get enough sleep had worse grades than those who got proper sleep.

- **Healthy Weight:** "Sleep and metabolism are controlled by the same sectors of the brain. When you are sleepy, certain hormones go up in your blood, those hormones drive appetite." – Dr. Rapoport

- **Avoid Depression:** A good night's sleep can help a person decrease anxiety. You get more emotional stability with a good night's sleep.

- **Improve Performance:** have less daytime fatigue and more stamina.

- **Sharpen Attention:** Study shows people who get less than eight hours of sleep were more likely to be inattentive and impulsive.

- **Spur Creativity:** people strengthen the emotional components of memory during sleep, which may help spur the creative process.

Good Posture – Good for Your Health! Poor posture distorts alignment of bones, chronically tenses muscles, and contributes to stressful conditions such as: loss of vital lung capacity, increased fatigue, reduced blood and oxygen to the brain, limited range of motion, stiffness of joints, pain syndromes, reduced mental alertness, and decreased productivity at home and work. – Paul C. Bragg, N.D., Ph.D.

Chapter 7

Bragg Back Fitness Program
with "Spine Motion" for a pain-free back

Oh! My aching back! This cry has echoed down the corridors of time for countless centuries, ever since humans learned to walk on their own two feet. This unique accomplishment – achieved only by human beings among all the varied forms of mammals on Earth – has given us the mobility and dexterity to cope with any environment found on Earth.

OUCH!

As with almost everything in nature and life, however, there is a price to pay for these accomplishments. Humans are still learning how to stand erect! From babyhood on, every human being repeats the slow learning process – crawler, toddler, walker, runner – and **all through life humans must pay attention to posture and maintain it, or suffer painful backache and its many related ills.**

Millions suffer with back pains needlessly! Today start your Bragg Back Program.

75

The Spine Is Your Vital Key to Health

Universal native folklore equates the backbone with courage, an intuitive tribute to erect posture and the key role of the spine in physical fitness. However, physical fitness is more than muscular power: It is the superior condition of the miracle human body and its frame.

When your body is fit and every muscle or organ is functioning properly, that body becomes a powerhouse of vim and vigor. Physical fitness means more than just plain health and the absence of illness: it means no hidden liabilities and no silent, painless illness working away like termites at the organic framework of your human house. **Remember, the spine is the ridgepole of your body – which is your earthly home and temple.**

Role of Spine in Miracle Human Body

Let us briefly summarize the key role of the spine in almost every function of the human body. It is the pivot of the skeleton – the framework of bones giving the body its shape. Anchored to the spine are layers of large and small muscles and ligaments of the back and abdomen, essential in holding the body erect and the vital organs in place (even these organs themselves are supported by the spine). In four-legged (*quadrupedal*) creatures, vital organs are suspended downward from a curved spinal column. However, in the two-legged (*bipedal*) human, they must be held up against the pull of gravity by an erect, strong spinal column.

In the center of the spinal column, descending directly from the base of the brain and protected by the bony vertebrae, is the miracle spinal cord, the control center of the extensive, intricate networks of motor and sensory nerves that radiate to all parts of the body (page 83).

For these basic anatomical and physiological reasons, (which we will discuss in detail during the course of this book), we believe that many ills can be traced to an abnormal spine. For example, prolonged habits of incorrect posture – as well as accidents, sudden movement, jolt or strain – can cause a vertebrae to shift slightly out of alignment (subluxation) and to press against a nerve passing out from the spinal cord through an opening at that level. Such an impingement is an open invitation to trouble in the organ or body part that is serviced by that partially pinched important nerve (see pages 83-86).

For similar reasons, the spine itself is often thrown out of alignment and into abnormal curves toward the sides, front or back of the body. This can adversely affect other bones of the skeleton, shorten or stretch muscles and ligaments, cause organs to prolapse (fall) and/or bring on interrelated painful malfunctions throughout the body.

Practice The Bragg Healthy Lifestyle, good posture, and these back and spine exercises. An ounce of prevention is worth a ton of cure!

Of all knowledge, that most worth having is knowledge about health. The first requisite of a good life is to be a healthy person. – Herbert Spencer

Body Misuse Causes Injury Over Time

It is estimated that as much as 80% of the population will experience back pain at some point in their lives. In fact, back pain is second only to the common cold as a reason for visiting a doctor. Annually, nearly 65 million Americans experience back pain, at a skyrocketing $150 billion yearly for medical treatments and disability payments, some on permanent disability!

According to Thomas G. Gutheil, M.D., Professor of Psychiatry, at Harvard Medical School, *"There are many reasons for an aching back, a number of which have to do with lifestyle changes, fitness, and the modern environment. Not only does the back carry the body, but it also carries many of the psychological tensions that humans get weighted down with. In my psychiatric training, I learned to look at the posture and body position for clues to a person's mental state: the stooped back whose owner seemed bowed by the weight of depression, the shoulders drawn in and tight, and the head retracted like a turtle's in anticipation of a blow that comes only in the fearful patient's imagination, and the many other posture giveaway signs."*

Sheila Reid, Rehabilitation Services Coordinator at the New England Spine Institute, observes, *"The single event that people think caused their back injury is often not the problem. Instead, it's almost a cumulative trauma. We go through years of back misuse and maybe years of an unhealthy lifestyle and then there is the one fall or the box or child you pick up that breaks the proverbial camel's back."*

The ratio of nerves sending messages about our backs, in comparison to the nerves on our fingertips, is much less than a hundred to one! Therefore, we are receiving fewer warning pain signals from our backs. Sad facts: most people tend to ignore their back until it starts crying out to them, calling for help to be relieved of pain and discomfort!

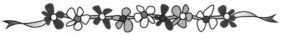

One study involving 12,000 back pain sufferers found that 80% enjoyed complete or significant improvement in symptoms after participating in a six-week program consisting of specially designed strengthening, relaxation and flexibility exercises. – Wellness Report, UC Berkeley

Bragg Originates Spine Motion Exercises

Modern machines are taking the place of manual labor, and have significantly deteriorated the physical body over the last 100 years. However, *Spine Motion* can help alleviate almost any back pain you may encounter and help keep it from decreasing your quality of life. In order to help alleviate back problems arising from structural spine problems, Paul C. Bragg originated the *Spine Motion Exercises* given in this book.

These spine exercises were introduced over 70 years ago. Public and press reception was so enthusiastic that claims made by those who used these exercises sounded extravagant. Only a small part of the amazing results reported would have to be true to establish the principle of *Spine Motion* as the valuable force that it is.

As remarkable as the results attained by you and others following these *Spine Motion Exercises* may be, we do not want anyone to regard this as evidence that these exercises can supplant all other health measures. They cannot, nor are they intended to do so. You must follow a well-rounded Healthy Lifestyle Program, including proper nutrition, adequate rest and other forms of exercise, all of which we will discuss in this book.

Spine Motion Exercises are also not to be considered a cure for any condition, illness or disease. In fact, nature has no cures, in a generally accepted sense of the word. **Your miracle body is self-healing and self-repairing when you work with Mother Nature, not against her! If one feels sick and miserable, it's usually brought on by your failing to obey her Natural Laws.**

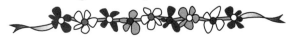

Remember: It's never too late to strive to be what you want to be! So start to Plan, Plot and Follow through! – Patricia Bragg

No wonder back pain is the second most common cause of missed work days, and the leading cause of disability between the ages of 19 - 60, and the number one impairment in occupational injuries. It is estimated 8 out of 10 people have back problems some time in their life. Please don't be one of these people!

Paul C. Bragg Recalls
Remarkable Results with Spine Motion

Bragg Spine Motion Exercises are a natural, drug-free approach to health. They are designed to help restore the spine to its natural, normal functions. This helps eliminate the causes of many apparent ailments in the back and other parts of the body that arise primarily from defects in spinal structure. These defects are brought on by poor posture, flabby muscles, improper living and bad working habits or accidents and injuries.

If you're under medical care, please consult your doctor on these exercises and the healthy lifestyle suggestions presented here. Many Orthopedists, Neurologists, Osteopaths, Chiropractors, Health Professionals, Physiotherapists and Acupuncturist (pages 231-234) find this program helpful to their patients.

I have seen back injuries and displacements (having resulted from slips, falls, coughs, sneezes or other sudden movements) respond wonderfully to these *Spine Motion Exercises*. Occupational accidents, such as sprains, strains or improper lifting, pulling, carrying or bending, often produce the type of pain and misery that *Spine Motion Exercises* can help relieve (see pages 101-111).

At one time, when I returned home from a Bragg Crusade, I found a relative in pain. He had been preparing a piece of ground to plant an organic vegetable garden, and had come across a large, heavy stone. Not realizing how heavy it was, he strained his back trying to lift it. Unable to continue his work because of severe, crippling back pain, he had been taking all kinds of treatments; however, the condition persisted. I advised him to take hot baths (*add 1 cup vinegar*) daily and, right after the bath begin very lightly doing *Spine Motion Exercises*. He followed my advice, doing the simpler exercises first, gradually progressing to the more strenuous ones. At the end of one week his pains were gone, and in another week he was once more working in his organic garden.

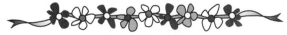

Nature, time and patience are the three greatest physicians.
– Irish Proverb

I have known cases of severe injuries to the back, such as whiplash from auto accidents, in which great relief was attained by lightly performing simple *Spine Motion Exercises*. I have also helped many athletes return to normal after a severe back injury, especially in physically punishing sports like wrestling and football.

A lifelong athlete myself, I have engaged in all types of sports and my daily practice of *Spine Motion Exercises* has strengthened my spine so much that I have never had any serious back injuries, despite some bad spills.

We have received letters and e-mails from people all over the world who have followed these exercise instructions and found pain relief from such conditions as lumbago, sacroiliac pain and postural defects of long duration. These exercises have also relieved painful cases of bursitis (inflammation of the bursa, especially of the shoulder, elbow and knee joints), sciatica, arthritis and persistent migraine headaches.

Millions Suffer from a Defective Spine

 Researchers have indicated that one in five sufferers of back pain are born with one leg longer than the other. This imbalance can put excessive pressure on the back and spine, the hips and knees.

About 1 out of 150 persons (of average development) has a sufficiently flexible spine. In today's society, the majority of people are sedentary, warping their spines by faulty posture in their sitting, standing and walking habits (page 69), along with lack of exercise and an improper diet! This applies not only to adults, but children and teens. Many schools no longer require basic physical education.

A study of teenagers in 7th and 8th grade, reported 11% with Scoliosis, or spinal curvature. The research was conducted among 841 students in Downey, California, by Dr. Leon Brooks, an orthopedic surgeon in the spine deformity service of Rancho Los Amigos Hospital. Dr. Brooks noted that untreated Scoliosis can be responsible for future back pains and respiratory problems! Special exercises are the basic treatment, except in severe cases requiring temporary back braces or, in extreme cases only, surgery.

Spine Motion is Simple and Scientific

Sporadic or incorrect work and exercise can take its toll on the spine, as can overly strenuous exercise, common among construction workers and some athletes. From the thousands of spine and back cases in our vast files, **here are three Spine and Back illustrative examples:**

The **first case** is a person whose spine was so badly slumped that it disturbed his nerve reflexes; he could not take part in ordinary youth sports. After only four weeks of *Bragg Spine Motion Exercises*, he became normally active. Later, he developed into a remarkable swimmer.

The **second case** is a logger in Northern California who, at age 55, was forced to abandon his rigorous outdoor work due to subluxation of the spine (partial dislocation of some vertebras). He started the *Bragg Spine Motion Exercises* and in less than a month, he was able to resume logging. Here was a man who for years had swung an ax, surely a vigorous form of exercise! Even so, the spine had become defective from lack of extension in the right directions and to the right degree. It required the peculiar, anatomical twist of the more scientific Spine Motion to align and flex his spine at every point.

The **third case** is of a 43-year-old woman who was clearly headed for invalidism, with organs supposedly far out of place and ailments that had defied ordinary forms of correction. After a few days of practicing the *Bragg Spine Motion Exercises*, she obtained complete relief.

The three cases just described are widely diverse, yet all three responded beneficially to the same *Spine Motion Exercises*. Why? Remember the spinal column is the focus of the neuromuscular and musculoskeletal systems. Even a slight dislocation or malfunction in the spine can affect other body parts and cause problems.

When recovering from accidents, fractures, etc. it's wise to take extra herbs, minerals, vitamins and drink distilled water to help body heal faster. – Dr. Linda Page • HealthyHealing.com

---

Researchers have discovered the more healthy habits an individual practices, the longer they live and the healthier and fitter they are!
– Elizabeth Vierck, Author of "Health Smart"

The Spine Works as a Miracle Machine

A Scientific Study of the Spinal Structure has made it possible to devise simple spine motions that give your miracle spine the requisite pull or stretch to restore its natural alignment and flexibility. Life holds many examples of what resilience means. Imagine an automobile without shocks, a trampoline without springs or a piano without felt hammers. In thinking of anything mechanical, just recall that every machine ever designed is patterned after the master mechanism constituting the human body. The more perfect the machine, the closer its designers have come to the principles of motion found in your miracle human body.

The effects of such motions have been carefully recorded and compared. It's been found that these simple manipulations, through careful, active use of the trunk muscles, cause all of the tiny bones comprising the spinal column to separate normally and build up the cushiony growths of cartilage between each pair of bones.

Spine Motion Helps Keep Spine Youthful

Miraculously, the cartilage responds readily to the stimulation of these *Bragg Spine Motion Exercises,* which are designed to stretch the spinal column and open the natural spacing between vertebras. Cartilage grows from the moment it's given room to develop. It's this quick restoration of cartilage (plus nutrition) that makes it astonishingly easy to accomplish apparent miracles with *Spine Motion Exercises*, irrespective of the person's age. In fact, age effects cartilage growth less than almost any form of replacement in the body. It's possible to produce abundant cartilage, and have a biologically youthful spine, regardless of your calendar years!

Let us now explain your spine (the body's mainspring) – its structure and function and how you can give it the loving care and attention it needs to fulfill its built-in potential of performing many years of good service for you.

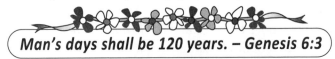

Man's days shall be 120 years. – Genesis 6:3

Chapter 8

Your Spinal Nerve System

The spinal cord is your body's vital "Control Center"

The most important function of the spine is to protect the spinal cord, the vital control center without which the musculoskeletal system and other vital organs of the body could not operate. Not even the most sophisticated computer system can match the performance of this cord of nerve tissue. Less than 12 feet long, little more than 3-inches in diameter and weighing about an ounce . . .

> **the spinal cord is the calculator and relay center of a vast and intricate miracle network of nerves that reach into every part of the human body!**

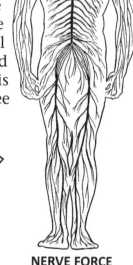

The spinal cord passes through the canal formed by the vertebral arches, continuous with and extending downward from the base of the brain (*medulla oblongata*). At the first lumbar vertebra, the single cord ends in a number of delicate filaments or threads that extend to the end of the spine and fasten the spinal cord to the coccyx. Cerebrospinal fluid maintains pressure in the cord, which is insulated from the bony canal by three layers of coverings called meninges.

83

THE NERVOUS SYSTEM IS THE COMMUNICATION SYSTEM OF YOUR BODY

Your Nervous System is made up of vital nerves which extend throughout your body and brain and vary noticeably in diameter.

NERVE FORCE

Our brains, every vital organ, every muscle, every cell of the body is directly governed by our nerves. – Paul von Boeckmann, early 1900's leading authority in America on breathing and nerve culture

Central Nervous System and Spine

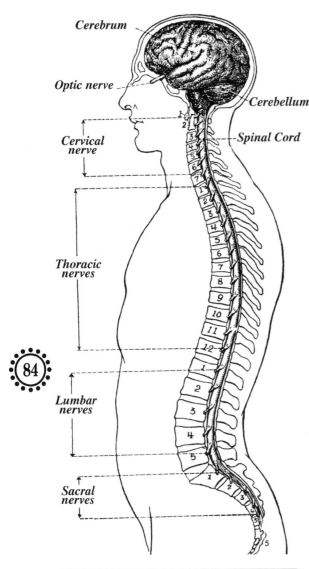

Cerebrum

Optic nerve

Cerebellum

Cervical nerve

Spinal Cord

Thoracic nerves

84

Lumbar nerves

Sacral nerves

VIEW OF CENTRAL NERVOUS SYSTEM & SPINE

It is in the cushions between the bones of the spine that the inorganic minerals and toxins from water may deposit themselves and cause backaches, slipped discs and many other health problems of the spine. Important nerve energy to vital organs may be greatly lessened which can cause many painful miseries throughout the entire body.

AREAS AFFECTED
by Spinal Subluxation

Vertebrae # . . . . . . .Affects

CERVICAL NERVE:

1-2 . . . . . . head, ears, eyes, sinuses, sympathetic nervous system

3-6 . . . . face, nose, lips, mouth

7 . . . . neck glands, shoulders, arm, hands, wrists, fingers

> headaches, dizziness, insomnia, allergies, high blood pressure, eye and ear problems, fevers, skin and gland problems, throat problems, thyroid, asthma, head colds, cough, numbness

THORACIC NERVE:

1-2 . . . . heart, lungs, breast

6-8 . . . . . . gallbladder, liver, digestive organs

9-10 . . . . . . spleen, adrenal

11-12 . . . . kidneys

> heart conditions, bronchitis, indigestion, heartburn, ulcers, allergies, hives, blood sugar, varicose veins, fatigue, low blood pressure

LUMBAR NERVE:

1-5 . . . . intestines

> gas pains, sterility, colitis, constipation, diarrhea

SACRAL NERVE:

1-5 . . . . . . sex organs, uterus, glands, prostate, bladder, knees, lower back

> cramps, hemorrhoids, impotency, poor circulation, pain/numbness/tingling, swelling from hips to feet

Miracle Spinal Nerves Control Our Actions

The spinal nerves pass through openings in the vertebral arches and branch out to serve various parts of the body. There are 30 pairs of these nerves: 7 cervical, 12 thoracic, 5 lumbar, 5 sacral and 1 coccygeal. Roots of the sensory nerves, which convey feeling, are attached to the back or dorsal side of the spinal cord. Roots of the corresponding motor nerves, controlling action, are attached to the front or ventral side. Each pair controls a specific part of the body. Example: if you stub your toe against a piece of furniture, the branch of the sensory nerve to that foot flashes a pain signal to the central control in the spinal cord, and the matching motor nerve immediately transmits the order to pull back the foot. This is done so swiftly that your reaction seems instantaneous.

Except for those controlled by the 12 cranial (brain) nerves, automatic or reflex actions are controlled by the spinal cord. For example, we *see* in our brain via the cranial optic nerve, but certain eye muscles are controlled from the spinal cord, and we *cry* by order of a spinal nerve that controls the lacrimal gland. Conscious actions naturally originate in the brain, but when these become reflex, they are usually transferred to the control center of the spinal cord.

In computer terminology, the brain *programs* a course of action and when it becomes habit it becomes part of the *database* of the spinal cord. When you learn to drive a car, for example, at first you must consciously think out every move, but with practice, it becomes automatic. Experienced drivers automatically calculate the speed of their own vehicle and other cars on the road, then decide how much acceleration will be required to pass safely. If they had to stop and figure this out consciously, they would never pass another car; but it's done in a split-second by their spinal nerve reflexes. The same thing happens in emergencies and in countless daily actions (like walking, sitting, etc.) programmed from infancy. Already in the database of our spinal computer at birth is its lifelong role in regulating breathing, heartbeat, circulation, digestion, elimination and reproductive functions – you are a miracle!

The Miracle Spine and Nervous System

Now you see why it's so important to keep your spine long, strong and flexible. It is made to protect your spinal cord and to stay in perfect alignment while also allowing freedom of flexible body movements in all directions.

Through our nerves we experience every physical pleasure or pain. The spine, when kept straight, strong, flexible and elongated, allows every set of nerves to function freely. The spine that has settled or shortened has less space between the vertebrae, crowding the nerves that pass through openings in the vertebral arches. This finally causes painful pressure on the bones and nerves.

When such impingement occurs in the upper cervical vertebrae, at the base of the head or upper neck, it may bring on headaches. Occurring an inch farther down, the eye muscles may be strained. In the thoracic area, pressure on nerves to the stomach and/or other digestive organs may cause malfunction or distress there. Farther down, impingement may affect bowels or kidneys. In fact, there's no body part that is not affected in some way by the spinal nervous system.

Your Reflexes – The Body's Miracle Watch Guard

Take a look at these responses that keep your body happy and humming:

- **SNEEZE:** When dust or other particles aggravate mucous membranes inside your nose, you let out a loud "Achoo!" to get rid of irritants.
- **BLINK:** When a tiny insect or speck of sand is flying toward your face, your eyelids respond by quickly closing to guard against eye injury.
- **SHIVER:** A drop in body temperature makes your muscles contract in a series of rapid, small movements that helps the body generate heat.
- **HICCUP:** Stomach irritations can cause diaphragm contractions that pull in air. The "hic" is the vocal cords closing to stop air from entering the stomach.
- **PUPIL DILATION:** The eyes' response when things get darker so as to let you see better. In bright light, pupils constrict to protect the retina from being damaged.
- **COLON & STOMACH:** Every healthy horse, animal and human has, at times, colon gas – a form of reflex. When you get bad bacteria or food poisoning in your stomach, your body cleanses by vomiting or diarrhea.

Muscles, Mind and Nerves Need to Rest

To *"Rest"* means freedom from activity, quietness and tranquility. It means peace of mind and spirit. It means to rest without anxiety or worry. Your rest should refresh your whole nervous system and entire body.

To properly rest and be still, it's also important to wear no restricting garments that might hinder your blood circulation. Are your shoes too tight? Your collar? Your hat? Your belt? Your watch? Your bra and undergarments?* Your stockings? If so, then you are not really resting when you sit still or lie down. The best rest is secured when you have loose or better yet wear little clothing. Any clothes and shoes you are wearing should be comfortably loose and never binding!

Tight Fitting Clothes Can Lead to Back Pain

Tight form-fitting clothes may be the trend now-a-days, but this may lead to nerve compression which is one of the main causes of back pain. It also may restrict the movement of your hip bones which enforces pressure on the spine and can result in severe back pain. These are some fashion trends to be wary of:

• **Skinny jeans** that grip around your waist, thighs, hips and calves cause strain in the joints and excessive nerve compression in your back muscles and may even cause a herniated disc and muscle problems.

• **Oversized handbags and shoulder bags** place more weight on one side of your shoulder. This can damage your back and may cause your spine to curve, which is one of the causes of back pain.

• **High heels** can cause calf muscles to shorten and throw off posture which may lead to blood circulation problems and back pain. Dr. Scholl says high heels throw the female organs off-balance (see page 116).

Tight brassieres should not be worn – they block proper lymphatic drainage in breast area and this can cause cancer.
– Dr. Doris Rapp, author of "32 Tips That Could Save Your Life"

**Read "Dressed To Kill," by Sydney Singer on breast cancer and wire bra studies.*

Nerve Energy is Essential to Health

Nerve energy is so essential to mental and physical health that we recommend you read more about it in our Bragg companion text, *Building Powerful Nerve Force & Positive Energy* (see back pages for book list).

Herein we are primarily concerned with the spinal column and its relationship to the part of the central nervous system that is controlled by the spinal cord. For peak performance of these nerves, which greatly influence the health of your entire body, a fully flexible, strong, healthy, elongated spine is vitally essential. *We believe in prevention.* Chiropractors are interested in helping you maintain a healthy spine and body! It's wise to have your spine checked from time to time by a chiropractor, who will help you with their specialized knowledge and training in displaced vertebrae and back and neck problems! A chiropractor will help you to keep your spine strong, healthy and in perfect alignment, if you do your part and keep the muscles strong and healthy by doing these *Spine Motion Exercises.*

88

See these websites on Chiropractic Therapy:
•*spine-health.com/treatment/chiropractic* •*SpineUniverse.com*

Health Road or Sickness Road?
Which Road Will You Take?

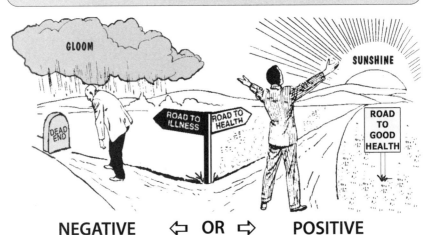

GLOOM

SUNSHINE

ROAD TO ILLNESS   ROAD TO HEALTH

DEAD END

ROAD TO GOOD HEALTH

NEGATIVE   ⇦ OR ⇨   POSITIVE

The choice of which road to take is up to you.

You alone decide whether to reach a dead end or live a healthy lifestyle for a long, healthy, happy, active life. – Paul C. Bragg

Chapter 9

Vitamins & Minerals
Vital for a Healthy Spine

Back pain due to faulty diet

Remember that the bones comprising your spinal column and the rest of your skeletal system are living tissue and must receive the proper nourishment in order to be strong and healthy for your entire long lifetime.

Your basic bone structure, as we discussed previously, consists of a rigid outer sheath that gives the bone its shape and strength, filled with elastic, spongy material called marrow. Engineers have adapted this structural principle in the construction of buildings, finding that supports such as metal pipes that are filled with dirt, for example, are stronger, more enduring and resilient than solid, rigid structures. Usually these man-made structures, however, deteriorate with time. This is not so with the miracle living bones of the human skeleton.

Our bones do not grow brittle only with age. They become brittle, weak and porous because of deficiencies in the diet. This condition is known as Osteoporosis, from *osteo* for bone, *por* for pore and *osis* for disease, a pore being a small hole like those through which we perspire.

Although Osteoporosis has long been considered an almost inevitable affliction of people over 50 years of age, the time element is not the basic factor. It is true that the longer you abuse your body by incorrect diet, inadequate exercise and insufficient rest, the greater price you will pay in the degenerative symptoms commonly known as ageing. However, this can happen at any stage of your calendar years! Look at the number of young men and women who are rejected from the armed services and from civilian work requiring good physical stamina, because of various physical deficiencies, from fallen arches to spine curvature and obesity, all due sadly, primarily to the habitual American fast food diet of dead foods, plus an unhealthy lifestyle!

Healthy Foods Prevent Osteoporosis

When we were doing nutritional research along the Adriatic Coast of Italy, we found ageless men and women, advanced in calendar years but whose bodies were youthful and supple and bones firm, strong and resilient. Their diet consisted primarily of organically grown fresh salads, properly cooked vegetables, olive oil, dark breads, pasta and natural cheeses rich in calcium, vitamins and minerals, all essential for strong bones. In our extensive research on nutrition, we rarely found osteoporosis among active people who lived on a simple diet of live, natural healthy foods (see more on page 28).

Your Spine Needs Organic Minerals

The only way to protect yourself against osteoporosis, or to restore weak, porous, brittle bones to a healthy state, is by proper nutrition! Given the proper tools to work with, the miracle body is self-healing and self-repairing, but don't expect overnight miracles. If you have been eating incorrectly for a period of time, it is going to take time to repair the damage after you make the change to a program of natural nutrition. Start today! Eliminate the dead foods from your diet, and give your bones and the rest of your body the live foods on which they can and will thrive.

For strong, healthy bones and a spinal column that really serves as the mainspring of your body, particular attention should be paid to the foods that supply the organic minerals essential to bone building. These are calcium, phosphorus, magnesium and manganese.

"While back pain can be structural, often the root cause is not your back, but rather an imbalance elsewhere in the body," says Dr. Sinett, NYC Chiropractor. He discovered a link between diet and back pain. His father, bedridden for nine months with back pain, then cut out sugar and caffeine from his diet. He gained his life back Sinett says, those foods elevate a person's level of cortisol, which is inflammatory in the body that can lead to pain. Imbalances elsewhere in the body such as digestion, emotions, or in your feet can create back pain. Also being overweight contributes to back problems and structural imbalance.
Dr. Sinett, author "3 Weeks to a Better Back" www.DrSinett.com

CALCIUM is important in reparation of all cells and the major component of the bones of the body. Ninety percent of the body's calcium is found in the skeletal system, where it's not only used as the main ingredient of bone structure, but also stored for use elsewhere in the body as needed! If your diet is deficient in natural, organic calcium, your bones will not only suffer from this lack, but they will become further weakened by the drain on their inadequate supply for other uses throughout the body. For example, during pregnancy the fetus draws on its mother's calcium supply, and if she is deficient, her teeth and bones suffer as do the child's.

Although only 1% of the body's calcium is used by the soft tissues, it is vital to health, especially of the nerves. It is not just the spinal column that needs this organic material, but also the spinal cord itself. Usually, the most noticeable sign of calcium deficiency is extreme nervousness. Without enough calcium in the blood, nerves have trouble sending messages. Tension and strain result; it is impossible for the body to relax. This is apparent in children who are highly emotional. It shows first by an unpleasant disposition, fretful 91 crying, temper tantrums, and sadly could develop into muscular twitching, spasms and even convulsions.

Calcium Deficiencies Affect All Ages

Both adults and children reveal calcium deficiencies by nervous habits such as biting the fingernails and restless body movements of hands, legs and feet (called restless leg syndrome), irritability and jumpiness. This calcium / magnesium deficiency can be a major contributing cause of adverse personality changes.

Fortunately, an adequate supply of calcium in the system has the opposite effect. In our years of experience and research, we have seen the meanest, most irritable, nervous people make personality changes for the better becoming happy, healthy, peaceful people, by following our Bragg Healthy Lifestyle of good nutrition and living habits! Also, calcium contains the natural material that causes the blood to clot when needed. If we did not have calcium in our bloodstream, we could prick a finger with a needle and bleed to death!

Calcium & Magnesium are especially important for healthy bones & heart.

Locations in the Body Where Osteoporosis, Arthritis, Pain and Misery Hit the Hardest

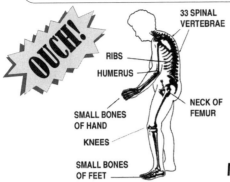

OUCH!

33 SPINAL VERTEBRAE

RIBS

HUMERUS

NECK OF FEMUR

SMALL BONES OF HAND

KNEES

SMALL BONES OF FEET

OSTEOPOROSIS
Affects over 60 Million and Kills 400,000 Americans Annually Estimated 50% of adults 65 years or older also suffer from Arthritis.

Boron: Miracle Trace Mineral For Healthy Bones

BORON – An important trace mineral for healthier and stronger bones that also helps the body absorb more vital calcium, minerals and necessary hormones! Good Boron sources are most organic veggies, fresh and sun-dried fruits, avocados, prunes, raw nuts and soybeans.

The U.S. Dept. of Agriculture's Nutrition Lab in Grand Forks, ND, says Boron is usually found in soil and foods, but many Americans eat a diet low in Boron. They conducted a 17 week study which showed a daily 3 to 6 mgs. Boron supplement enabled participants to reduce loss (demineralization) of calcium, phosphorus and magnesium from their bodies. This loss is usually caused by eating processed fast foods, drinking tap waters (distilled is best), eating lots of meat, salt, sugar and fat and a dietary lack of fresh vegetables, fruits and whole grains. (*all-natural.com*)

Scientific studies show women✱ benefit from a healthy lifestyle that includes vitamin D3 sunshine and exercise (even weight-lifting) to maintain healthier bones, combined with distilled water, low-fat, high-fiber, carbohydrates, and fresh organic fruits, salads, sprouts, greens and vegetable diet. This lifestyle helps protect against heart disease, high blood pressure, cancer and many other ailments! I'm happy to see science now agrees with my father who first stated these health truths in the 1920's.

92

✱ *For more hormone and osteoporosis facts, read pioneer, Dr. John Lee's book – "What Your Doctor May Not Tell You About Menopause"*

Boron helps keep the skeletal structure strong by adding to bone density, preventing Osteoporosis, treating Arthritis and improving strength and muscle mass. Boron helps facilitate calcium directly into the bones. Boron protects bones by regulating Estrogen function. Boron is naturally found in beans, nuts, avocados, berries, plums, oranges and grapes. Boron helps relieve menopause symptoms and PMS. – Dr. Axe

Natural calcium sources (page 94) offer a wide variety of important minerals you can include in every meal. Protein foods high in calcium, for meat eaters, include: organ meats like liver, kidneys, and heart; natural, unprocessed yellow cheeses; fresh, fertile eggs. Stone-ground cornmeal, whole natural oatmeal and whole natural barley are fine sources; so are raw nuts and seeds. Green leafy vegetables abound in calcium, alfalfa sprouts, spinach, beet greens, mustard greens, collards, broccoli, kale, cabbage, cauliflower, dandelion greens, lettuce, also snow peas, carrots and cucumbers. Fruit sources include: oranges, sun-dried dates, figs, prunes and raisins.

Milk is Not the Best Source of Calcium

Most Americans believe milk is the best way to get the calcium your body needs, but there are many reasons why this is not true (see web: *notmilk.com*).

First: almost all American milk is both pasteurized (boiled) and homogenized to kill any bacteria that might make you sick! This process also reduces the available calcium in milk.

Second: milk also contains an enzyme called lactose to which most people are allergic! The major symptom of lactose intolerance is mucus formation, but most people don't recognize this symptom as the allergic response that it is.

Third: you must take into the account the herbicides, pesticides and fungicides that cattle ingest through their foods, and the hormones, growth stimulators, antibiotics and other drugs that are pumped into cattle to treat disease and maximize weight and milk production. All of these toxins are passed on to you through their milk. *Avoid dairy products and fulfill your calcium requirements with these nutritious foods in the chart on the next page.*

Triticale (hybrid cereal grain) has zinc, phosphorous, manganese and calcium, all integral parts of bone production and strength in the body. Adding Triticale to your diet can significantly boost bone growth, speed up bone healing and prevent conditions like osteoporosis.
– www.OrganicFacts.net

Calcium Content Chart of Some Common Foods

Calcium Food Source	mgs	Calcium Food Source	mgs
Almonds, 1 oz	80	Kale, (raw/steamed) 1 cup	180
Artichokes, (steamed) 1 cup	51	Mustard Greens, 1 cup	138
Beans, (kidney, pinto and red)	89	Oatmeal, 1 cup	120
Beans, (great northern / navy) 1 cup	128	Orange, 1 large	96
Beans, (white) 1 cup	161	Prunes, 4 whole	45
Blackstrap Molasses, 1 Tbsp	137	Raisins, 4 oz.	45
Bok Choy, (steamed) 1 cup	158	Rhubarb, (cooked) 1 cup	105
Broccoli, (raw/steamed) 1 cup	178	Sesame Seeds, (unhulled) 1 oz	381
Brussel Sprouts, (steamed) 1 cup	56	Soybeans, 1 cup	73
Cabbage, (raw/steamed) 1 cup	50	Soymilk, fortified, 1 cup	150
Cauliflower, (raw/steamed) 1 cup	34	Spinach, (raw/steamed) 1 cup	244
Collards, (steamed) 1 cup	152	Tofu, firm $1/2$ cup	258
Corn tortilla	60	Turnip greens, 1 cup	198
Figs, (5 medium)	135	Whole wheat bread, 1 slice	17

Sources: Back to Eden, Jethro Kloss; Health Nutrient Bible, Lynne Sonberg; **website:** www.vrg.org/nutrition/calcium.htm, chart by Brenda Davis, R.D.

PHOSPHORUS combines with calcium, vitamins A and D in proper proportion for balanced bone structure and body metabolism. *Natural Phosphorus Sources* include: all organ meats; fish and cod-liver oil; natural cheese; raw spinach, cucumbers, alfalfa sprouts, peas, kale, mustard greens, watercress; brazil nuts; whole-grain rye, whole wheat, bran; and raw wheat germ.

MAGNESIUM is necessary for calcium and vitamin D metabolism which help to build and prevent the softening of bones. *Natural Magnesium Sources* include: stringbeans, peas, garbanzos, kidney beans, dried lima beans; Brussels sprouts, chard, cucumbers, alfalfa sprouts, raw spinach; bran and whole wheat; avocados; pine nuts and sunflower seeds; prunes and raisins; and honey.

MANGANESE is an important trace mineral that serves as a carrier of oxygen from the blood to the cells. It is particularly important in the nourishment of the intervertebral discs and cartilage that have no direct blood circulation. *Natural Manganese Sources* include: fish, poultry, liver, fertile egg yolk, organ meats, all natural cheese; dulse, sea kelp; potatoes – especially the skins; lettuce, watercress, celery, onions; alfalfa sprouts, peas, all beans; bran and organic cornmeal; almonds, filberts, chestnuts, walnuts; and bananas.

Remember that your body must have natural organic minerals (i.e., from plants and living sources). Neither humans or even animals can assimilate inorganic rock minerals, as they come directly from the earth. Only plants can digest inorganic minerals into an organic form that can be used as food by animals and humans.

So, if you take mineral supplements, make sure these are from organic sources! To take inorganic calcium tablets, for example, would not supply your bones with the calcium it needs; it would only clog up your system with indigestible chalk! Health Stores have natural supplementary organic sources of calcium and other organic minerals essential for strong, healthy bones.

Vitamins Essential to a Healthy Spine

All-natural vitamins are important for health. Of special importance to a healthy spine are vitamins A, C and D for building and maintaining strong, resilient bone structure. The B-complex vitamins are especially essential to the spinal cord and the nervous system.

VITAMINS A & D: are essential in regulating the use of calcium and phosphorus – the two major elements in the formation, building and maintenance of bones – in the body. Vitamins A and D are also vital to the efficient functioning of the nervous system. They act together as catalysts in this important phase of body metabolism. Without them, the parathyroid glands of the endocrine system cannot carry out their primary function of maintaining the balanced interaction and distribution of calcium and phosphorus, and both bones and nerves deteriorate. There is a marked drop in bone density in people whose diet has been deficient in vitamins A and D over a period of time. Abnormal spaces appear in the bone structure, and the bone cells become thin, brittle, and almost looks like swiss cheese: this is Osteoporosis.

An important strategy for healthy bones is to eat the right kind of foods. A diet full of processed foods will produce biochemical and metabolic conditions in your body that will decrease your bone density, so avoiding processed foods is definitely the first step in the right direction. – www.mercola.com

Natural sources of vitamin A are colored fruits and vegetables such as carrots, yams, yellow squash, papaya, apricots, peaches, melons and dairy products (we avoid), fertile eggs, liver, fish and cod liver oil.

Natural sources of vitamin D include fish, cod liver oil, unsaturated fats, fresh fertile eggs, organic milk and butter, but **the prime source is sunshine.** A daily gentle sunbath (before 10 am or after 3 pm) will supply your quota of vitamin D, as well as improve your health in many other ways. Give your body time to absorb vitamin D through the skin before washing off perspiration after a sunbath.

VITAMIN C: supplies collagen, the adhesive that holds together all the cells in the bones, nerves and body tissues. Without Vitamin C, we would literally fall apart. Since the body does not store this powerful antioxidant, we need a constant supply of vitamin C in our daily diet. ***Natural sources of C*** are citrus fruits, berries, greens, cabbage and green bell peppers. These should be eaten raw and fresh, since cooking easily destroys vitamin C.

VITAMIN B1: Thiamin Chloride – often called the anti-neuritic or anti-beriberi vitamin, aids growth and digestion and is essential for normal functioning of the nerve tissues, muscles and heart. Deficiency signs include nervous irritability, fatigue, insomnia, loss of weight and appetite, weakness and lassitude and mental depression.

VITAMIN B2: also called Riboflavin, promotes general health and particularly affects the health of the eyes, mouth and skin. It is important for growth and red blood cell production. Riboflavin works as an antioxidant, fighting free radicals. Deficiency is often evidenced by itching, burning or bloodshot eyes, inflammation your of mouth, a purplish tongue and cracking of mouth corners.

VITAMIN B6: Pyridoxine, is a water-soluble nutrient that prevents various nervous and skin disorders. It helps support adrenal function and aids in food assimilation, protein and fat metabolism. Nervousness, insomnia, and loss of muscular control are signs of it's deficiency.

VITAMIN B12: Cobalamin, *a great energy vitamin,* aids in the important formation and regeneration of the red blood cells (produced in bone marrow) and is essential in prevention of anemia, osteoporosis and heart disease. It also promotes growth in children, and is an energy tonic for adults, especially seniors! Deficiency may lead to pernicious anemia, growth failure and poor appetite in children and seniors and also the diseases above.

VITAMINS B-COMPLEX: It's important to include the entire B-Complex in your diet, and nature has provided for this. Nutritional yeast heads the B12 foods list, followed by raw wheat germ and fertile eggs, especially egg yolks; fish; and natural cheeses. Natural, unsalted peanut butter (not hydrogenated) is an excellent source of B-Complex; also raw or freshly roasted peanuts. Non-GMO whole grains: barley, 100% whole-grain flours, buckwheat flour, cornmeal and organic oatmeal and rice husks. *Vegetable sources include:* raw and dried beans like lima, soybeans and green beans; raw and dried green peas; leafy vegetables, collards, kale, turnip greens, mustard greens, spinach, broccoli and cabbage. B-rich fruits are oranges, grapefruit, bananas, avocados and cantaloupe. Blackstrap molasses is a good source. Alone or with other dishes, mushrooms add B-vitamins.

VITAMIN K1 and K2: Work synergistically with calcium. A biological role of Vitamin K2 is to help move calcium into proper areas in the body, such as the bones and teeth. It also helps remove calcium from areas where it should not be, such as your arteries and soft tissues. In a nutshell, it's important to maintain a proper balance between calcium, Vitamin D and K2 as well as magnesium. *Sources of Vitamin K1 and K2:* Vitamin K1 is found in vegetables and Vitamin K2 is found in relatively few foods – organ meats, egg yolks and Japanese Natto. Also you can take K2 supplements – 1,000 mcg a day.

We take natural vitamins and mineral supplements as our added insurance for super health! Be sure they are from organic, all natural sources (no soy, gluten, preservatives, GMO or dairy) that are best for your health.

- How can I stop inorganic minerals and chemicals from hardening and turning my brain and body into painful calcification, stiffness and stone?

- How can I stop my body's joints and back from becoming painful, stiff and cemented?

- How can I help stop the formation of gallstones, kidney stones and bladder stones?

- How can I protect my arteries, veins and capillaries from the unnatural, hardening of arteriosclerosis?

- How can I prolong my health and youthfulness?

- How can I prevent sickness and premature ageing?

The answer is to live The Bragg Healthy Lifestyle, eat healthy foods and drink pure distilled water!

Jack LaLanne Became Healthy, Youthful and Ageless – You Can Be Too!

98

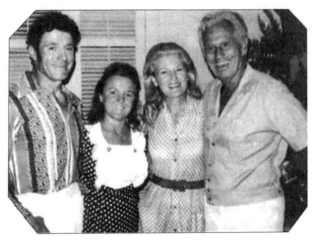

Jack LaLanne, Patricia Bragg, Elaine LaLanne & Paul C. Bragg

Jack says he would have been dead by age 16 if he hadn't attended The Bragg Health Lecture. Jack says, *"Bragg saved my life at age 15, when I attended the Bragg Health and Fitness Lecture in Oakland, California."* From that day on, Jack faithfully lived *The Bragg Healthy Lifestyle*, inspiring millions to health, fitness and a long and happy life! See his website: *www.JackLalanne.com*

Chapter 10

Stretching the Spine Promotes a Healthy Back and Body

Stretches to avoid the stretcher

As we noted earlier, you are *taller* when you arise in the morning, because a relaxing night's sleep allows your spinal column to stretch. Why doesn't it stay this way through the day? Why the need for special exercises?

Ordinary activities of the average person, from student to executive, housewife to movie star, simply do not use the spine to its full amazing capacity! Nature constructed the human spine to withstand an enormous amount of activity, constant use and even abuse. It is this very endurance that renders the ordinary activities, and even strenuous ones, inadequate for stretching the spine. Years of walking, riding, sitting, bending, turning, lifting and carrying have all made your spinal column so accustomed to bodily exertion that it is scarcely extended beyond the extremities of normal movement.

To a degree, Nature does replace the cartilage lost by constant wearing down, but there is rarely sufficient stretch of the spinal column in daily activities to separate the vertebrae the required amount. A little ground is lost each day, as in the case of Nature's restoration of tissue, blood, bone or anything else; this is, essentially, what is known as the process of ageing or *growing old*.

Nothing, of course, can bring the process of ageing to a 100% full stop. Unfortunately, most humans accelerate it by working against Mother Nature, failing to obey her laws. As we have discussed, the spinal column is a key factor in practically all of our life processes. That is why *Spine Motion Exercises* will not only stretch your spine, but also stretch your life in years and in the living of those years to the full enjoyment of vigorous health and vitality.

Natural Spine Motion

Animals practice natural Spine Motion. For example: watch a dog or cat arching their back that spreads the vertebrae. A cat will lower the forepart of its body (page 111), extending its forepaws far forward and often will twist their head and shoulders. This natural Spine Motion is the chief reason why these animals have such unabated energy over so long a portion of their lives. A dog whose normal life is eleven years, for example, will not show any noticeable ageing signs until its eighth or ninth year, and some will stay youthful until they are into their teen years.

Spine Motion Exercises Benefit Entire Body!

Many such bonuses come from these *Spine Motion Exercises*. By scientifically stretching your spine, you will at the same time strengthen the muscles and ligaments supporting it, thus helping to hold the spine elongation and greatly improving your posture. Circulation and nerve energy will be stimulated throughout your body. Digestion will improve, as pressure on controlling nerves is relieved, and as organs become more firmly supported in correct position. You will breathe deeper, giving your body cells more of that priceless invisible food, oxygen.

Make Every Spine Motion Exercise Count

When you first start limbering up the back, you may have some muscle soreness, but don't stop exercising. After a few days of continuous daily periods of exercise, muscle soreness will disappear. **Soon, you will find great satisfaction in doing these spinal exercises and the beneficial effects will amaze you.** Now, let's get started!

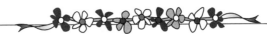

Keep Healthy and Youthful Biologically with Spine Motion Exercises and Good Nutrition.

You will increase your energy, joy, peace of mind, and improve your health, (sleep too) with more daily exercise and deep breathing.

Here Are Five Bragg Spine Motion Exercises:

Now, let's get started with the five main *Bragg Spine Motion Exercises*. Each one is different in effect, though they all effectively stretch your spine for better health. Take a momentary rest between each one, but do the entire series.

Spine Motion Exercise #1

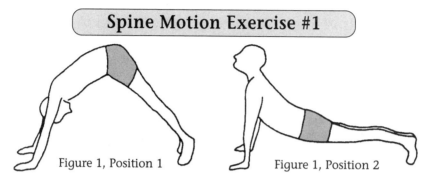

Figure 1, Position 1   Figure 1, Position 2

This first *Spine Motion* applies specifically to the nerves that affect the head and eye muscles. A reflex of the same motion affects a set of nerves that go to the stomach and bowels. Thus, in one movement, we attack eye strain, headache, indigestion and poor assimilation.

Lie face down on the floor. Now, rise to an arched position in which you rest on your hands and toes with the back highly arched (see Figure 1, Position 1). The pelvis will be higher than the head. Feet are spread about 15 inches apart. The knees and elbows must be kept stiff.

Now, drop pelvis almost to the floor (See Figure 1, Position 2). **Remember: keep elbows and knees stiff (this is essential to impart the proper spinal stretch).** As you lower the back, gently bring your head back; raise it as you lower the body. This is not a fast motion; take your time in execution. Dip to extreme low, then rise high again, arching the back all you can; down again, then up, and down. If you do this motion correctly, you will find that a few times are enough. **If only you could see what is going on along the spinal column during this jackknife action, you would know the relaxation and great relief imparted to the nerves all along the spine.**

Spine Motion Exercise #2

This second *Spine Motion* is designed to stimulate the nerves leading to the liver and kidneys. It can bring relief from many of the nervous conditions that are manifested in subnormal functioning of these vital organs. A sluggish liver and nonelastic kidneys, prematurely aged, for which there is no real excuse, will respond with surprising swiftness to this spinal torque or twist. This exercise helps quickly bring these organs to a healthier state of vigorous function.

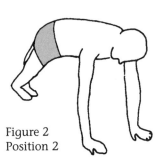

This motion starts in the same arched position as #1 (Figure 1, Position 1): face down, weight resting on hands and toes, back highly arched, with elbows and knees stiff.

Figure 2
Position 2

Now, swing the pelvis slowly from one side to the other, to the very limit of your ability in each move to the right, then to the left, back and forth (Figure 2, Position 2). This motion should be done slowly. Always think of the s-t-r-e-t-c-h we must give the spinal column.

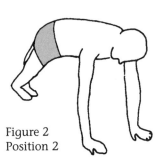

At first, you will find this motion tiring. It will grow steadily easier to do, not so much because of muscular development, but rather because of vastly improved nerve organization. It should never become perfectly easy. This is more than a simple swaying of your body; you must make every one of long row of vertebraes stretch away from those adjoining them.

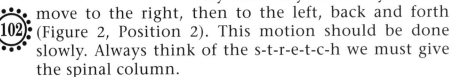

Your Daily Habits Form Your Future

Habits can be wrong or right, good or bad, healthy or unhealthy, rewarding or unrewarding. The right or wrong habits, decisions, actions, words or deeds . . . are up to you! Wisely choose your habits, as they can make or break your life! – Patricia Bragg, Health Crusader

The natural healing force within us is the greatest force in getting well.
– Hippocrates, Father of Medicine, 400 B.C.

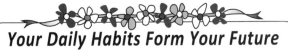

Be your own Health Captain and do what needs to be done for your health!

Spine Motion Exercise #3

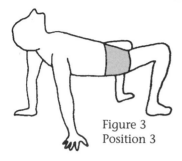

Figure 3
Position 3

In this third *Spine Motion,* the entire spinal column is flexed from top to base. Every nerve center is stimulated. The pelvic region is specifically helped. This motion also strengthens those muscles attached to the spine that are most helpful in retaining the vertebrae in this improved and elongated position, that stimulates the growth of the intervertebral cartilage.

Take a new starting position for this motion. Sit down on the floor; then, raise the pelvis up by placing hands at sides (palms down) and drawing in the feet about 12 inches. You are now resting your weight on the flats of your hands and feet, with pelvis and back up off the floor.

Raising the body, let the spine be horizontal as you finish the upward movement (see Figure 3, Position 3). Now, go down to the starting position, but lowering yourself to just above the floor. Go up once more, then down. Two of the many remarkable benefits are the strengthening of the muscles and the spine.

Follow These Tips for a Strong Healthy Back

Physicians confirm that stretching your spine is imperative for everything from prevention of injury to flexibility and strength. Murray C. Oransky, M.S., P.T., writes, *"The back muscles should be stretched daily, along with all muscle groups around both hips, as these muscles connect to the back,"* and he stresses the important relationship for us between our daily lifestyle habits and back pain.

You may be using your back muscles improperly, or making these common mistakes: 1. standing in one position for prolonged periods of time without elevating one leg (resting one foot on phone book or low stool) 2. bending over to pick something up without bending at the hips and knees 3. bending over to pick something up and twisting back while bending or 4. carrying objects awkwardly too far away from the body.

People who follow healthy living habits in early adulthood spend less time coping with disability in the years before their death. – Stanford University

Spine Motion Exercise #4

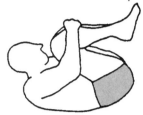

Figure 4, Position 4

The fourth *Spine Motion* brings a particular force to bear at the curve of the spine where the nerves affecting the stomach are clustered. This motion also has the greatest efficiency of the whole series in actual lengthening of the spine from top to bottom. The miracle results are felt in overall improvement. After all, it is the general stretching of the entire spinal column that brings the whole system to top balanced efficiency.

Daily upon awakening lie on the bed or on the floor on your back, hands at your sides. Bend your knees and bring to chest position, clasping arms around your legs a few inches below your knees. Now pull your knees and thighs tightly against your chest. At the same time, raise your head and try to touch your chin to your knees (Figure 4, Position 4). Hold this squeezing position for at least five seconds. Relax and then repeat exercise.

104

Spine Motion Exercise #5

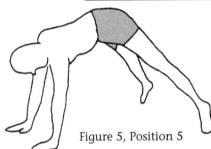

Figure 5, Position 5

In addition to its spine-stretching benefits, this fifth *Spine Motion* brings speedy relief to sluggish bowels and organs both by nerve stimulation and exercise to the colon.

Assume Position 1 (page 101) lying face down on the floor, then rising to arched position, resting on your hands and toes, the back highly arched up, pelvis higher than the head (Figure 5, Position 5). Now, walk all around on all-fours. This baby-crawl exercise on knees and hands also helps tone the stomach and core muscles, especially after childbirth.

See famous book, "Stretching," by Bob Anderson, World's top Stretching Coach and Bragg follower. His wife did these sketches. Bob also gives Bragg Breathing Exercises at his Sports Seminars. www.stretching.com

Exercise How Many Times and How Often?

The number of times you do each of these *Spine Motion Exercises* will rest with you individually. At first, three to five times for each *Spine Motion* will extend you amply. In a day or two, increase the count to five times or more. Since these motions are entirely new, you might experience some muscular stiffness during the first few days; this will pass. After it does, when the spine, muscles and ligaments become more limber, a normally strong person will find ten times for each exercise no more difficult than were the three times of the first day.

How long to continue this series of *Bragg Posture and Spine Motion Exercises?* In the beginning, your spine-stretching routine should be a regular daily program. After you show marked improvement, two to three times weekly usually is sufficient to keep spine flexible.

Some people report that the very first session with *Spine Motion Exercises* has brought every apparent benefit promised, but it usually requires a week to see and start to feel the change. It is two to three weeks before the ground gained begins to take hold and assumes permanence of effect. **Remember your spine is a miracle!**

Please bear in mind the settling down process of the spine has been a matter of years. It is not a condition you can overcome in a day. It takes time, and these *Spine Motion Exercises* give the spine time to stay stretched and they stimulate cartilage growth and healing. Faithful daily practice of these exercises allows growth of cartilage under favorable conditions, thus securing the widened spaces between the vertebrae for a more healthy spine.

Staying in shape pays, partly because aerobic activity promotes circulation. If you already have back problems, the right kind of regular exercise, yoga, etc. will help prevent you from getting more severe pain and further injury.
– Stephen Hochschuler, M.D., Orthopedic Surgeon, Co-founder and Chairman, The Texas Back Institute, Plano, Texas

Types of Vertebrae

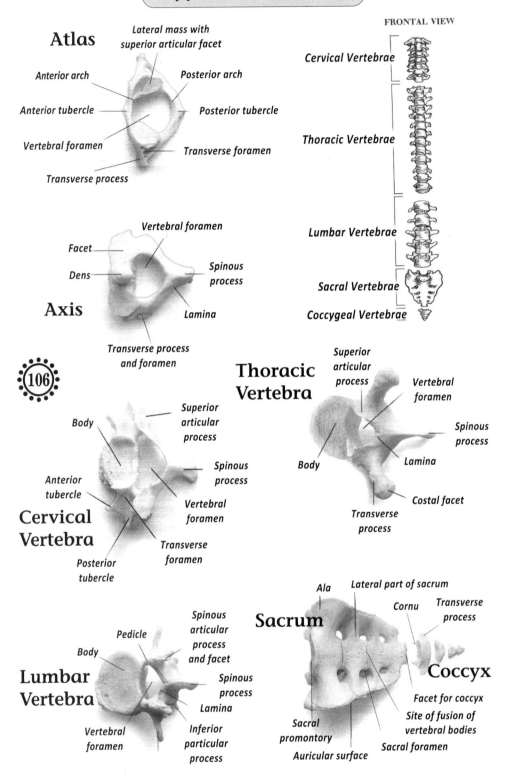

Atlas

Lateral mass with superior articular facet

Anterior arch

Anterior tubercle

Vertebral foramen

Transverse process

Posterior arch

Posterior tubercle

Transverse foramen

FRONTAL VIEW

Cervical Vertebrae

Thoracic Vertebrae

Lumbar Vertebrae

Sacral Vertebrae

Coccygeal Vertebrae

Axis

Vertebral foramen

Facet

Dens

Spinous process

Lamina

Transverse process and foramen

106

Cervical Vertebra

Body

Anterior tubercle

Posterior tubercle

Superior articular process

Spinous process

Vertebral foramen

Transverse foramen

Thoracic Vertebra

Superior articular process

Vertebral foramen

Spinous process

Lamina

Body

Costal facet

Transverse process

Lumbar Vertebra

Pedicle

Body

Vertebral foramen

Spinous articular process and facet

Spinous process

Lamina

Inferior particular process

Sacrum

Ala

Lateral part of sacrum

Cornu

Transverse process

Coccyx

Facet for coccyx

Site of fusion of vertebral bodies

Sacral foramen

Sacral promontory

Auricular surface

Chapter 11

12 Spine Motion Strengthening Exercises
Strengthening physical therapy exercises

In addition to the unique *Bragg Spine Motion Exercises,* here are some of the basic physical therapy exercises recommended by top Orthopedists for strengthening the spine and its supporting muscles. We have selected a healthy dozen to include in this Spine-Fitness Program:

#1   Neck Extension to Strengthen Upper Spine

Stand in correct posture position, feet apart, muscles relaxed. Clasp hands behind head. Lean head forward, then attempt to push it backward as you resist with your hands. Do this for six seconds, counting one-thousand-one, one-thousand-two, etc. Repeat with head straight up, then with head as far back as gently possible. Gently stretch your neck as far as you can in each direction.

#2   Back Stretching and Back Strengthening

This exercise gives wonderful relief whenever your back feels tired. Stand up and stretch, feet slightly apart, rising on your toes and reaching upward with arms, then relax. Now bend over at the waist, knees slightly bent. Hold your legs with your hands behind the knees. Pull in your stomach muscles and attempt to straighten your back, while resisting back extension with your hands. Hold for six seconds, counting one-thousand-one, one-thousand-two, etc. Then relax, stretch and relax again.

#3   Leg Extension for Strengthening Back

Lean over a table, palms of hands flat on top near edge, elbows bent, standing far enough away so head and torso bend comfortably parallel to table top, spine straight. Keep knees relaxed, feet flat on floor. Now, slowly raise one leg backward up high as possible. Hold for six seconds, counting one-thousand-one, etc. Slowly lower leg to starting position. Repeat with other leg. Continue, alternating legs, but stop when you begin to tire.

#4 Neck Rolling to Strengthen Upper Spine

Stand in a comfortable correct posture position with no tension. Now, bring your chin to your chest, roll your head to one side (trying to make your ear touch your shoulder), continue roll toward your back (stretching the neck gently back far as possible), rolling on to other side (trying to touch that shoulder with that ear), then rolling head back to starting position. Do this exercise slowly, s-t-r-e-t-c-h-i-n-g the neck muscles, 20 times from right to left, then 20 times from left to right. This exercise is a must for desk workers and helps relieve muscular tension in the neck and keep the cervical vertebrae extended.

#5 Rag Doll Exercise to Strengthen Entire Spine

Stand in a comfortable correct posture position, feet about 18 inches apart. Pretend your arms are those of a rag doll, completely limp, letting them bounce limply as you swing your body from one side to the other, turning with each swing to look as far back as you can over each shoulder.

#6 The "Old Favorite" Spine Bending Exercise

Stand erect with feet together. Raise hands over head, arms straight. Keeping the knees relaxed, bend forward and try to touch your toes with your fingertips. Gently stretch your torso downward to reach as far as possible, then return to the starting position. Next, with arms upraised, bend backward gently as far as possible, stretching the spine in the opposite direction. Return to starting position. Do this exercise at least 10 times.

#7 Spinal Twisting Exercise

Stand in a comfortable correct posture position, feet shoulder width apart. Extend arms to shoulder height at your sides. Holding arms in position, twist your body from the hips as far as possible to the right, letting your eyes follow the back of the right hand, then as far as possible to the left. Try to see the same thing directly in back of you when twisting to each side. Alternating right to left, repeat 20 times.

#8   Endurance Test to Strengthen Lower Spine

Lie flat on your back on the floor, arms at your sides. Keeping the knees stiff, lift your heels two inches off the floor and try to hold your legs and feet off the floor in this position for 60 seconds, counting one-thousand-one, etc. Each time you do this exercise, add a few more seconds. This really gives strength to the lower spine and is a wonderful workout!

#9   Hip Rolling to Strengthen Lower Spine

Lie flat on your back on the floor, arms extended at sides at shoulder height, feet together. Raise the right leg vertically, toes pointed upward, knee straight, then swing, roll leg over left, touching toes to floor beyond fingertips of left hand. Return leg to vertical position, then lower it to floor. Repeat same exercise with left leg beyond fingertips of right hand. Do this exercise 20 times, alternating right and left legs.

#10   On-Side Exercise for Strengthening Spine

Lie on the floor on your right side, legs straight, arms comfortable. Keeping the knee stiff, raise your left leg straight up, then return it slowly to starting position. Now, bend the knee and bring your left thigh up against your chest and try to touch your chin to the knee. Do this ten times on the right side, then turn over to the left side and repeat ten times with the right leg.

#11   Arm-Hanging Spine-Stretcher

If you have access to a door or wall bar, do this exercise from a rung high enough for feet to clear floor. If not, use a door that is fully open and steady so it cannot swing, and place a towel over top edge so you can get a good grip. Now, grasp top of door (or rung of bar) and relax your body, letting it hang down free. If you use a door, bend your knees so your feet will be off the floor. Remember, this is an exercise for your back, not your arms, so make your body dead weight to s-t-r-e-t-c-h your spine. Hang like this for few minutes, then relax briefly and repeat it at least three times.

#12 Shoulder Rolls for Cervical Vertebrae

Stand in a comfortable correct posture position, feet apart. Roll your shoulders way up, then as far forward as possible, then down, then as far back as possible. Do this 12 times in smooth, continuous circle motion. Pause briefly, then reverse circular rotation 12 times: up, back, down, forward. Increase daily from 12 to 30 times each way.

Take Exercise Breaks Throughout the Day

The first seven of these *Bragg Spine-Strengthening Exercises* can be done anywhere and anytime. All sedentary office workers should get up from time to time, stretch and do at least one of these exercises. You will return to your work refreshed with renewed energy. Instead of losing time, you will save it because you can work faster and better after an exercise recharger!

Dr. Henry L. Feffer, Professor of Orthopedic Surgery at George Washington University School of Medicine stated: *"The greatest strain on the intervertebral discs occurs while sitting, especially in an over-stuffed chair. The pressure per square inch on a disc is about twice as great when sitting as when standing, and this pressure is more likely to injure a disc if it doesn't have a good external muscular support, which is often the case in a sedentary person."* Dr. Feffer also stated: *"Usually the chair that an office executive gives his secretary is much better for the back than the swivel chair he uses himself."*

If you are a sedentary worker, as millions of Americans are, use a chair that helps you maintain correct posture at all times. Be sure to get up out of that chair (correctly) at intervals to stretch your spinal column and strengthen your muscles. Get off the elevator several floors below your own and walk up the final flights of stairs, head and chest up, spine in perfect alignment. Don't pull yourself up by the handrail; it's best to lean forward and up, pushing yourself from one stair to the next by the springy leverage of your hips, legs and feet.

❀ *Old age is not a time of life. It is a condition of the body.* ❀
It's not time that ages the body, it's abuse that does! – Herbert Shelton

Even if your work involves physical labor, remember that it is not necessarily the amount of exercise you do, it's the way you do it that counts. Remember the case of the *lumberjack* who *chopped* his spine out of alignment! If the muscles on one side of your spinal column are developed more than on the other, the spine can be pulled into a side curvature. Take time for exercises that *balance* those muscles of your body required in your work.

If your daily activities are primarily those of running a household, home or office you will find your day easier and less fatiguing if you use some of these exercises during your day. Also, take *breathers* at intervals to stretch and tone your spine and strengthen any unused muscles.

Sadly many schools don't require regular Physical Education classes. Teenagers and college students who have *outgrown* vigorous childhood games and recreation need to make a daily habit of practicing good posture and spine exercises. Spines can begin to *settle* even in teens!

The Healthy "Cat Stretch" Exercise

(111)

Among the Orthopedic exercises recommended in his book *Orthotherapy,* Dr. Arthur A. Michele, former professor and chairman of the Department of Orthopedic Surgery at New York Medical College and director of Orthopedic Surgery at 8 other NYC hospitals, is a healthy spine-stretcher that deserves special attention. Although Dr. Michele called it *Long Body Stretch*, we call it *Cat Stretch** because it reminds us of our cat's natural Spine Motion.

Kneel on floor with knees 6-8" apart. Keeping your thighs perpendicular to floor, bend forward from waist, stretching arms forward along the floor, let forehead drop down as though to touch floor, your torso sloping down from hips to elbows. Now, lower chest as close to floor as you can, pressing down for a count of 10. Return to starting (sloping) position for a count of 5. Repeat as many times as you can in 3-5 minutes. This exercise stretches the entire spine and also limbers up the shoulder joints.

*Cats are graceful, coordinated and instinctively stretch to keep muscles tuned and joints flexible. Notice how cats feel the stretch, test the tension, relax and focus on the stretch.

We have all seen animals, from cats to dogs to horses, lie on their backs and roll and wiggle their backbones with joy in soil or on the grass. According to another Orthopedist, Dr. Lloyd Kingsbury, they are not merely scratching their backs; they are exercising their spines. He adapted this spine exercise for humans as follows:

Lie on back, knees bent, feet about 18 inches apart, arms extended on floor at shoulder height, elbows bent with forearms parallel to head. Press the small of your back (lumbar vertebrae) flat against the floor, inching your hips downward, while your shoulders and head stretch back as your spine stretches out! Hold your body in this *natural traction* position as long as comfortable (count 1 to 20), relaxing when muscles begin to tire. Whether you feel tired or your back aches from physical or sedentary labor, these Spine/Back Exercises help give wonderful, refreshing spine-stretching relief.

Avoid Back Punishment – Protect Your Back

The single event that people think caused their back injury may not be the problem. *"Instead, it's almost a cumulative trauma,"* warned Sheila Reid, Rehabilitation Services Coordinator at the New England Spine Institute. *"We go through years of misuse, then there's one thing you lift or a fall you take that breaks the proverbial camel's back."* Even bowling, tennis or golf (all predominantly one sided sports) can cause back problems.

A heavy shoulder bag can punish your back, too. *"Putting extra weight on your shoulders unbalances your body and to compensate, many people twist their spines,"* says Rehabilitation Specialist, Dr. Karen Rucker of Virginia Commonwealth University. *"It's best to take out the things you don't need!"* This holds true also for shopping bags.

Long car rides can harm your back as well. The culprit is the phenomenon of whole body vibration. *"It's a risk factor for lower-back pain,"* said Dr. Malcolm Pope, a founding member of The International Society for the Study of the Lumbar Spine. Simple steps to take are: when the road gets rough, slow down (speed generally magnifies effect of bumps), stop to stretch every 2 hours on long drives. Upon arrival, rest fatigued muscles for a few minutes before unloading bags.

Chapter 12

Self-Care and Prevention, Put Your Back into It!

Use your "Backbone" for physical fitness

In carrying out this program of physical fitness with *Spine Motion*, you must use your backbone, in both senses of the word! In the folklore sense, of courage and willpower, you must use your backbone to transform your pattern of life from one of merely tolerable existence to living in full joy of radiant health! Particularly in the beginning, you will need mental discipline and willpower to reprogram your lifestyle habits of diet, posture and physical exercise in accordance with the natural laws of health and fitness, we have outlined for you.

Vital in this transformation is the exercise of your backbone: stretching and strengthening your spinal column with these unique *Bragg Spine Motion Exercises,* and easy-to-do posture and back strengthening exercises. Faithfully follow the instructions we have given you.

Do the exercises in this book slowly and gently for first week or so. At first, feel your way along so as not to get your muscles sore with overly vigorous contractions. Always exercise short of the point of pain. No matter what, don't stop your daily routine! A slight soreness is natural when your muscles have been unused, but it will disappear when you continue your program!

Remember: if you can move a muscle, you can strengthen it. We have never seen anyone who could move a muscle and was willing to really exercise daily yet couldn't develop a limber and supple spine, gain added strength, have a more active life, look and feel better and get more real enjoyment out of daily living!

Don't forget: if you don't use your spine, you will lose it. It will become prematurely old, stiff and painful. The body and spine remain youthful, supple and strong only with sufficient use, exercise and a healthy lifestyle!

You Are as Young or Old as Your Spine Is

No matter how you have neglected and abused your spine, by following the instructions given in this book, you can reverse the condition. **The recuperative powers of the human body are tremendous! The body is a self-repairing and self-healing miracle.** You must give your body the natural health aids it needs. When the correct nutrition and exercises are provided, you help your spine to repair and restore itself to strong health.

Within a few weeks of following the *Bragg Spine Motion Program* outlined, your spine will feel more flexible and supple. You will walk with a spring in your step. You will feel the vital energy surging through your body. You will be surprised how wonderful you feel when your spine limbers up! You will find you do not tire as easily. You will have more go-power and energetic drive.

It will not stop there. Each day, you will add new zest, vigor and power to your body. **Remember: the world is alive, you're alive; you are never too old to feel youthful and enjoy an ageless powerful body!** Now, get started and really begin to feel fully alive again! Like thousands of others, you will get a new lease on life as you follow The Bragg Healthy Lifestyle with this Back Fitness Program with *Spine Motion*. Life is sure to be enjoyed when your spine and body function perfectly.

114

The Miracle Spine-Brain Connection

Our spinal column and nervous system control everything in our bodies, from standing, sitting and sleeping to even using the bathroom. As our brain controls our body, our body sustains and revitalizes our brain by providing vital nutrients, oxygen, glucose and neurotrophins (nutrients which sustain neurons). These nutrients all travel through cerebrospinal fluid that flows inside the spinal canal. This fluid moves from the spine to the brain by the use of a "pump," which is powered by movement of the sacrum (lowest) and the cervical (highest) parts of the spine.

Miracles can happen every day through guidance & prayer! – Patricia Bragg

In order for the cerebrospinal fluid pump to work correctly, a healthy spinal column is needed. Damage, misalignment, and imbalance of the spine will result in an ineffective "brain-body connection." When impeded, the flow of these nutrients to the brain are also impeded, resulting in damaged brain tissue and function. Ultimately, this means there is increased risk of disease and the brain will begin to atrophy and deteriorate even before the age of 25! (*mercola.com*)

Orthotics Help Reduce Back Pain

The majority of lower back pain is not caused by direct injury – instead, it is the result of abnormal gait and repetitive motion injuries. Our precious feet are the body's foundation and every step that we take plays a key role in the absorption of impact and shock. Problems that result from our feet can radiate up to our knees, hips, and back. Sometimes, one can notice that lower back pain seems to increase when wearing certain shoes; this may mean that the feet are contributing to the pain!

By correcting the problems in our feet, we can improve our overall posture and lower-body alignment! Things like back, neck, knee and hip pain can be banished along with troublesome shin splints, all with the help of proper Orthotics to support the arch! Flat and high arched feet especially benefit from Orthotics, and Dr. Scholl's Foot Cushions (*DrScholls.com*) as they provide structure and relief for plantar fascia tissue along the bottom of feet.

Studies indicate you could also be at increased risk of Osteoarthritis if one of your legs is longer than the other – a condition that affects one in five Arthritis sufferers and can put excess pressure on the hip and knee of the side with the shorter leg. Experts say that chronic back or leg pain is one clue that your leg length may be off. Your doctor can measure it precisely, and a simple heel lift or Chiropractic adjustment may be all that is needed to correct it.

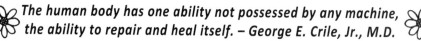
The human body has one ability not possessed by any machine, the ability to repair and heal itself. – George E. Crile, Jr., M.D.

High Heels Can Cause Pain & Wreck Health

Women should wear high heels with caution, and then only for special occasions! Low-heeled shoes are the best choice for day-to-day wear as they keep heels flat to the ground, much like walking barefoot as Mother Nature intended. High heels force the whole body forward, causing the back to curve in, the stomach to protrude and muscles in the legs to shorten. Women's female organs suffer from being tilted and off balance while walking in high heals (*on their toes and balls of their feet*). This is your body's way of compensating for being thrown off balance, but it can result in mounting aches and pains from your toes to your back and neck.

How to Handle a "Back Pain Attack"

Even though back pain comes on suddenly, there are factors leading up to an episode of pain that are cumulative and gradual. Things like poor posture, obesity and a weakened back and abdomen muscles. When muscle spasms hit, the first thing people want to do is lie down and rest for a while. This does reduce pressure on affected areas and permits inflamed tissue to settle down. Some people find that lying on one side with legs bent and a pillow between the knees provides optimal relief. Also rub Arnica on the area then pat on DMSO, see page 123.

Other ideas to help alleviate a "back pain flair-up":

TRY HEAT OR ICE: Either or both may help! You should wait at least 48 hours after an acute injury before applying heat, but otherwise, hot packs, hot water bottles or heating pads are advisable. Also sitting in a whirlpool or hot tub with apple cider vinegar is soothing. Heat dilates blood vessels, improving flow of nutrient and oxygen-rich blood to affected tissues. An ice pack is known to reduce inflammation. Although cold may feel painful against the skin, it numbs deep tissue pain. Applying either heat or cold may bring temporary pain relief, but will not cure the underlying cause of chronic back pain.

DON'T OVERDO BED REST: Short-term bed rest is fine, but studies have shown that too much bed rest can actually make matters worse. It's important to get up and start moving around as soon as possible. Be as active as you can be – usually after a day or two.

GET RELIEF WITH EXERCISE: Walking (pages 57-64), swimming, stretching and gentle yoga may help ease your pain.

MASSAGE MAY PROVE HELPFUL: Study found that the standard relaxation massage, also known as Swedish Massage (page 234) helped relieve back pain by stimulating tissues and calming the central nervous system.

Special Acupoints of the Spine

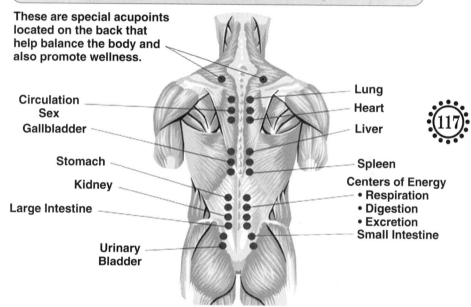

These are special acupoints located on the back that help balance the body and also promote wellness.

Circulation
Sex
Gallbladder

Stomach

Kidney

Large Intestine

Urinary
Bladder

Lung

Heart

Liver

Spleen

Centers of Energy
• Respiration
• Digestion
• Excretion
Small Intestine

(117)

Design created by David Carmos, Ph.D., from "Acupuncture and the Natural Healing Arts of the Far East" and "You're Never Too Old To Become Young" by David Carmos, Ph.D. and Shawn Miller, D.C.

When you are ready to start exercising again:

• Stretch! – Flexibility exercises all help to keep your muscles pliant.
• Keep up your core strength – the stronger your core, the more support you have around your spine and disks, the less likely to cause spasms.
• Watch your posture – slumping or standing in ways your body is not meant to, can invite micro-irritations. – Dr. Oz

What is Acupressure?

Acupressure is an ancient healing art that uses fingers to press key local points on the skin's surface to stimulate the body's natural self-curative inner healing abilities. When these points are pressed, they release muscular tension reaching also to the body's trigger points to promote healthier blood circulation and increase the vital life force to aid healing. Acupressure is the most effective method for self-treatment of tension-related ailments by using the power and sensitivity of the touch of the human hand. See web: *www.acupressure.com*

How Acupressure Can Help Relieve Pain

One of the popular alternative therapies available to help relieve back pain is *Acupressure*, which is often described as Acupuncture without needles. Acupressure is a system of massage that promotes the life energy, stimulating meridian points whether needles or fingers are used (see Acupoints of the Spine page 117).

Acupressure You Can Do Yourself

Foremost among the advantages of Acupressure's healing touch is that it's safe to do on yourself and others – even if you've never done it before – just follow the instructions and go gently and slowly! There are no side effects from this and the only equipment needed are your own two hands. You can practice Acupressure Therapy any time and anywhere, on friends, family and yourself! The Acupressure points are areas on

Exercises that strengthen your abdominal muscles, such as gentle sit-ups or crunches, help support your back. Please begin any exercise program slowly. – Berkeley Wellness Report

Life isn't about finding yourself. Life is about creating yourself. – George Bernard Shaw, Nobel Prize Winner in Literature, 1925

Dr. Sinett believes in listening to the whole body. There are three different levels: STRUCTURAL (muscles and bones); CHEMICAL (diet and nutrition); and EMOTIONAL (everyday stress). These three levels are at the core of what true health is all about. – Dr. Sinett • www.DrSinett.com

the body that are sensitive to the body's bioelectrical impulses. When you stimulate these points, it triggers the release of natural endorphins. As a result, pain is blocked and the flow of blood and oxygen to the affected area is increased. This causes the muscles to relax and promotes healing.

Besides relieving pain, Acupressure can help rebalance the body by dissolving the tensions and stresses that keep the body from functioning smoothly and which inhibit the immune system. Trouble-making tension tends to concentrate around Acupressure points. Along with Acupressure, you can use a combination of the self-help methods given in this book that can help improve your overall health and you will feel more alive, healthy, and in harmony with your life.

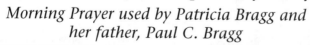

Morning Resolve To Start Your Day

I will this day live a simple, sincere and serene life; repelling promptly every thought of impurity, discontent, anxiety, discouragement and fear. I will cultivate health, cheerfulness, happiness, charity and the love of brotherhood; exercising economy in expenditure, generosity in giving, carefulness in conversation and diligence in appointed service. I pledge fidelity to every trust and a childlike faith in God. In particular, I will be faithful in those habits of prayer, study, work, nutrition, physical exercise, deep breathing and good posture. I shall fast for a 24-hour period each week, eat only healthy foods and get sufficient sleep each night. I will make every effort to improve myself physically, mentally, emotionally and spiritually every day.

Morning Prayer used by Patricia Bragg and her father, Paul C. Bragg

Get organized, be self-disciplined to live a healthy, long, fulfilled life.

PILATES is a complex gentle form of exercises and stretches – a fusion of Western and Eastern Philosophies, teaching you about breathing with movement, body mechanics, balance, coordination, positioning of the body, spatial awareness, muscle strength and flexibility. – Pilates.com

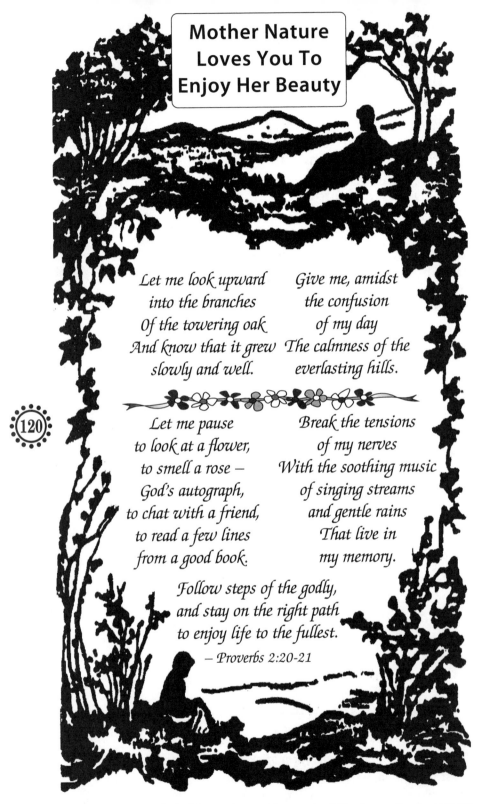

Mother Nature Loves You To Enjoy Her Beauty

Let me look upward
into the branches
Of the towering oak
And know that it grew
slowly and well.

Give me, amidst
the confusion
of my day
The calmness of the
everlasting hills.

Let me pause
to look at a flower,
to smell a rose —
God's autograph,
to chat with a friend,
to read a few lines
from a good book.

Break the tensions
of my nerves
With the soothing music
of singing streams
and gentle rains
That live in
my memory.

Follow steps of the godly,
and stay on the right path
to enjoy life to the fullest.
— Proverbs 2:20-21

Open your eyes to behold wondrous things out of Thy law. – Psalm 119:18

Chapter 13

Common Causes and Treatments for Back Pain

Back pain is an epidemic

The back and spinal system are so complex that it's often difficult to pinpoint the exact cause of back pain *(researchers have found strong links between a sedentary lifestyle and weak stomach/back muscles and chronic back pain)*. Add this to the many different approaches to understanding what is wrong, as well as the variety of options for addressing back problems, and you have a whole wide world revolving around the common experience of back pain felt worldwide!

This is true in America, where there is so much variety available in back treatments. The less industrialized countries often have fewer patient complaints about back pain – not because people don't suffer from it, but because it's considered part of every day life and they are not aware of it as a specific medical condition that can be diagnosed and cured. In contrast, backaches are the second most common reason for doctor visits in the United States (cold and flu are first). And for all the available treatments for Americans, they are generally dissatisfied with the medical care they receive. *"When something hurts, we want it fixed – and fast,"* says Bill McCarberg, Founder of the Chronic Pain Management Program for Kaiser Permanente in San Diego. *"It's frustrating to visit the doctor and find out, in most cases, the doctor can't solve the problem."*

"Our lives are in our smart phones," is often echoed throughout the high-tech world we live in today. With the different Health Apps, wearable sensors, and a little record-keeping, you can collect information such as food habits, nutrition, body measurements, sleep statistics and more. You can use this info at your doctor's visits so it can help you reach your well-being and health goals.

<u>Here are a few Health Apps you can download for free:</u>

• *MyFitnessPal: Set daily calorie goals, track food intake and exercise*
• *Kardia: Easy to use portable EKG, Detects AFib, FDA cleared.*
• *Sleepbot: Track sleep, then get a wakeup call when sleep is lightest*

In spite of the difficulty in pinpointing the cause and best treatment of back problems, years of research and experience have lead the medical community to the following knowledge: *"I think we can say with certainty now that bed rest and traction are bad ideas,"* says Daniel Cherkin, Scientific Investigator at Washington Health Research Institute. *"They both can weaken the muscles supporting the back and make problems worse."* Most researchers also agree that only between 2% to 5% of back patients really require surgery, and only for cases of tumors, spinal fractures, and extreme leg pain due to nerve compression in the spine. Beyond these, it's up to each individual to seek and discover the best approach that works for them! For this reason, be familiar with alternative therapies, such as: chiropractic, acupuncture, acupressure, exercise, massage, and yoga. See back pages for a list of Alternative Therapies (pages 231-234).

Pulled Back Muscles, Strains and Sprains

A *sprain* is defined as an injury in which a ligament (the tough fibrous tissue that connects bones to other bones) is stretched or partially torn. A *strain* occurs when a muscle or tendon (the tissue that connects muscle to bone) is stretched beyond its normal range. It can be difficult sometimes to determine whether you have a strain or a sprain. Both may result in painful muscle spasms, as well as bruising, swelling and painful movement. It doesn't matter if it is a muscle strain or a ligament sprain that is causing the pain, since the treatment for both is the same.

Fortunately, back muscle strains usually heal with time, most healing within a few days and almost all resolving within 3 to 4 weeks. The large muscles in the lower back have a good blood supply, which provide the necessary nutrients and proteins for healing to take place.

The more mechanically out of alignment a person is,
the less energy is available for thinking, metabolism and healing.
– Dr. Roger Sperry, won Nobel Prize in Physiology and Medicine, 1981

A good laugh, walk & long sleep are the best cures in the doctor's book.

Treatments for Pulled Muscles & Sprains:

MASSAGE: which can help promote blood flow in the lower back (to help healing), loosen tight lower back muscles, and release endorphins, the body's natural pain killers.

CHIROPRACTIC: Gentle manipulation to help loosen tight back muscles and promote healing in lower back.

COLD PACKS OR ICE: helps reduce inflammation. Also, pat Arnica and then some DMSO – it's helpful after injury.

HEAT THERAPY: Applying heat to lower back is helpful longer term to stimulate blood flow to the injured area.

If an episode of lower back pain lasts for 2 weeks, muscles may start to weaken. Because using lower back muscles is painful, the natural tendency is to avoid using them. However, the lack of activity leads to disuse atrophy (muscle wasting) and subsequent weakening, which in turn can cause more lower back pain because muscles are less able to help hold up the spine.

The Radiating Pain of Sciatica

Sciatica is pain that originates in the lower back area and radiates down one thigh to below the knee, usually into the foot. The pain is often persistent and more severe than a "run-of-the-mill" backache. It can also be accompanied by numbness, tingling and/or muscle weakness. It is estimated that four in ten people will experience it at some time in their lives.

Often Sciatica is caused by a bulging or herniated intervertebral disc that irritates or compresses a spinal nerve root. Also Spinal Stenosis (the narrowing of the spinal canal) can cause Sciatica in people over 50. Another possible cause is Piriformis Syndrome. This occurs when the Piriformis muscle deep in the pelvis goes into spasm or becomes inflamed and presses on the Sciatic nerve.

 For most people Sciatica typically gets better on its own and healing process usually takes a few days to a week.
— *www.SpineHealth.com*

Natural Treatments for Sciatica include:

Alternative remedies and regular exercise will go a long way toward relieving the pain most people experience.

HEAT/ICE: can help alleviate leg pain, especially in the initial phase. Usually ice or heat is applied for approximately 20 minutes, and repeated every two hours. Most people use ice first, but some find more relief with heat. The two may be alternated. It is best to apply ice with a cloth or towel placed between the ice and skin to avoid an ice burn.

CHIROPRACTIC THERAPY: Spinal adjustments and the manual manipulation performed by chiropractors and osteopathic physicians, are focused on providing better spinal column alignment to help address a number of underlying conditions that can cause Sciatic nerve pain.

ACUPUNCTURE: This practice is centered on the philosophy of achieving or maintaining well-being through an open flow of energy via specific pathways in the body. Hair-thin needles (usually not felt) are inserted. Acupuncture has been approved by the U.S. Food and Drug Administration (FDA) as treatment for back pain, and the National Institutes of Health have recognized Acupuncture as effective in relieving back pain, including Sciatica (more info on Acupuncture pages 118 and 231).

COGNITIVE BEHAVIOR THERAPY: taking control and lifestyle changes can be helpful in managing Sciatica pain, particularly in the short term. Sessions with a therapist may be face-to-face or online.

MASSAGE THERAPY: has been shown to have a number of benefits for back pain, including increased blood circulation, muscle relaxation, and release of endorphins, the body's natural pain relievers (see more info on page 234).

This list represents most common treatments, but is by no means comprehensive. There are many more options, and patients will often need to use a process of trial and error to find out what works best for them.

Technology to Treat Sciatica

Millions of lower back pain cases are related to disc problems. If a bulging disc is pressing on a spinal nerve root, the pain can radiate into the leg causing Sciatica. Two minor procedures are available to help with this type of back pain:

Intradiscal Electrothermoplasty (IDET): This simple procedure involves the insertion of a needle into the affected troubled disc with guidance of an X-ray machine. A wire is then threaded down through the needle and into the disc until it lies along the inner wall of the annulus which is the outer-shelled disc. The wire is then heated which destroys small nerve fibers that have grown into cracks and have invaded degenerating disc causing pain.

Radio-frequency Discal Nucleoplasty: with this minimally invasive procedure a needle is inserted into the disc, and a special radio-frequency probe is inserted through the needle into the disc. This probe generates a highly focused plasma field with enough energy to break up the molecular bonds of the gel in the nucleus, essentially vaporizing some of the nucleus. The result is that 10-20% of the nucleus is removed which decompresses the disc and reduces the pressure both on the disc and surrounding nerve roots. This procedure may be more beneficial for Sciatica type of pain than IDET, since Nucleoplasty can actually reduce disc bulging which is pressing on a nerve root. The high-energy plasma field is actually generated at relatively low temperatures, so danger to surrounding tissues is minimized. For info *www.SpineUniverse.com*

"Fortunately for mankind, the back has developed so well that it's capable of withstanding stresses and strains better than many other parts of the body. There are some who insist the back is the weakest part of man. Actually, it is one of the strongest. If it could be given the same amount of personal consideration and attention we give regularly to the teeth, the skin and other portions of the body that are more easily visible, the human back and body would be a more efficient mechanism and would last much longer without breaking down."
– Dr. Morris Fishbein, Journal of the American Medical Association

What is a "Slipped Disc?"

The chief shock absorbers of the spinal column and the *ball bearings* that give it such great flexibility and resilience are the intervertebral discs. These little cushions between the vertebrae are composed of a *stuffing* of extremely elastic tissue. The tissue is the consistency of a pudding, but very tough, called the Nucleus Pulposus, which is encased in a laminated (layered) covering called the Annulus, resembling an onion but exceptionally tough and resilient. It is reinforced at the top and bottom by the Cartilage Plates, which protect the disc from contact with the bones.

When the spine flexes, the discs are compressed in that direction, pushing the nucleus in the opposite direction to fill the extra space between the vertebrae. In strong, healthy spines, the *ball bearing* function of these discs can withstand a great deal of pressure. However, if the Annulus (covering) becomes weakened, or if the disc is subjected to severe compression by a sudden accident, jolt or undue strain, the pressure on the nucleus pushes it through the outer covering into the spinal canal. In medical terms, this is called a Ruptured Intervertebral Disc or Herniated Nucleus Pulposus (known as a *slipped disc*). When this occurs, the disc is pushed (*slipped*) out into the spinal canal.

A slipped disc blocks the passageway and produces damaging pressure on the spinal cord. At the same time, the adjoining vertebrae, robbed of their cushion, then press against each other and on the nerves coming out from the spinal cord. Until this injury became so prevalent during World War II, primarily from bouncing in jeeps over rugged terrain, the resulting severe pain was frequently diagnosed as Sciatica or other forms of lower back pain. Once the true cause was discovered, however, remedial surgical techniques were developed. These have now become so perfected, that practically normal spinal function can be restored. In addition to avoiding sudden or severe strains, the best way to avoid a future slipped disc is to lengthen and strengthen up your spine with our *Spine Motion Exercises*, good posture and healthy nourishment, so that your discs will be strong, healthy, tough and resilient.

The medical approach to disc problems is often a combination of painkillers, muscle relaxers, and physical therapy. It may involve hot or cold packs, baths, traction, electrical stimulation, laser and as a last resort, surgery.

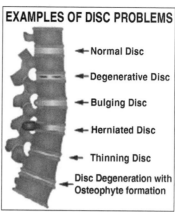

EXAMPLES OF DISC PROBLEMS

- Normal Disc
- Degenerative Disc
- Bulging Disc
- Herniated Disc
- Thinning Disc
- Disc Degeneration with Osteophyte formation

The first steps to deal with herniated disc problems are conservative. These include bed rest, analgesics, chiropractic and physical therapy. At this point it's prudent to have x-rays done in search of indirect evidence of a disc problem, and to see if any degenerative changes exist on the spine. If these measures fail, then a possibility of surgery may be contemplated, based on examinations using an MRI (magnetic resonance imaging) or CT scan (computer tomography) to show the disc or any rupture and the space behind it and the nerves. The EMG (electromyography) shows nerves and muscles. If you do suffer from a slipped/herniated/ruptured disc, first consider a natural alternative before you consider surgery!

Alternatives to Painful Back Surgery

Our 23 spinal discs help give our spine its sideways curves (a curved spine is 16 times stronger than a straight one) and also join the vertebraes together. Discs contribute to our height – in the morning we are about $1/4"$ – $1/2"$ taller than we were the night before because our discs thin a little during the day and expand a little while we sleep. The discs themselves don't actually *slip*, since they are knitted into the vertebrae from above and below. What sometimes do slip are the vertebrae, which may put pressure on the disc and contribute to its damage. Many *slipped discs* would be more accurately called *slipped vertebrae*. Since regular x-rays cannot *see* a disc, an MRI or CT scan is necessary to reveal any disc problems! Ironically, it's not unusual to find people with no pain show herniation, even ruptured discs, while others with pain show no disc problems at all. This demonstrates the complexities of spinal pain.

Advantages of Spinal Cord Stimulation

Finding effective treatment for chronic back and neck pain, can be very challenging. When surgery or other treatments have been unsuccessful or are not an option, Spinal Cord Stimulation (SCS) may offer relief and improved daily functioning. The medical literature has shown that Spinal Cord Stimulation is potentially effective for a number of chronic pain conditions, such as back pain, neck pain, and complex regional pain syndrome, that have not been helped by other treatments. Unlike most surgical procedures, Spinal Cord Stimulation Therapy is reversible. If a person decides to discontinue the Therapy, the electrical contacts, wires, and generator can all be removed and there are no permanent changes to the spine.

Spinal Cord Stimulation Advantages:

ADJUSTABLE PAIN RELIEF: Pain varies widely from person to person, and even with the individual at different times. Having control over pain can be a welcome change for those dealing with a chronic condition.

MINIMALLY INVASIVE PROCEDURES: There is typically just one incision needed – to implant the generator – and even-smaller generators do not require long incisions. It has few side effects and is easily reversible; if it doesn't work or is no longer needed it can be removed.

REDUCED OPIOID USE: Pain relief experienced with SCS may allow people to take fewer pain medications.

TARGETED PAIN RELIEF: Instead of taking a medication that affects the whole body and causes sleepiness, constipation, or other problems unrelated to the pain, SCS delivers pain relief only where it is needed.

LIMITED OR NO SIDE EFFECTS: Doesn't have the type of side effects associated with many medications.

COST-EFFECTIVE PAIN RELIEF: Researchers have found that the costs associated with SCS compare favorably with alternatives, including non-surgical treatments.

 Prevention is always preferable to the cure.

Vertebral Disc Regeneration

The upright adult spine loses up to ¾ of an inch of vertical height each day due to a loss of fluid from the vertebral disc. While our normal sleep cycle allows the unloaded discs to re-hydrate by absorbing the fluid surrounding the discs, not all of it can be fully recaptured. This is why, by age 60, it's common to lose up to 2" of stature. For quite some time it was presumed by the medical field that once a spinal disc had degenerated and lost its height, that it could not be restored; and furthermore, that such degeneration was not preventable. Not true!

Before learning how to reverse and prevent vertebral disc degeneration, first the causes of this degeneration must be addressed! Our spinal discs are composed of 88% water; when the body dehydrates, the first place it pulls water from is the "white tissues" which are the ligaments and tendons of our body, including the vertebral discs. A loss of only 12% water leads to a 50% reduction in disc height! Please stay hydrated!

> **The intervertebral discs need three things to re-hydrate and regenerate: motion, water and nutrients.**

To allow for re-absorption of spinal fluid, consecutive alternating compression and traction of the discs will allow the discs to "suck" the water back in from the cerebrospinal fluid. Following these special exercises, one must allow for plenty of water and proper nutrition, focusing on a bone strengthening diet and lifestyle.

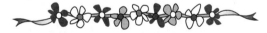

Spinal Cord Stimulation does not eliminate all pain, but has the potential to significantly reduce pain. For more info: www.SpineHealth.com

Stem Cells may ease back pain. Dr. Todd Gravori, Neurosurgeon & Director, ProMed Spine in Beverly Hills, CA, states that he has experienced success in using Stem Cells to stop progression of degenerative disc disease. "As technology becomes more sophisticated and doctors learn more about what these cells are capable of, treatment for spinal conditions will be revolutionized." – For more info: ProMedSpine.com

New Technology: Disc Regenerative Therapy

Disc Regenerative Therapy or DRT, is an exciting procedure that triggers the body's natural healing mechanisms, relieving pain and often curing the cause. DRT promotes healing through injection of a glucosamine and dextrose solution into the center of the disc. These natural substances stimulate growth of new collagen fibers and increase the strength of the painful disc. The procedure takes about 30 minutes, without risk of surgery, general anesthesia or hospital stays, and without a prolonged recovery period. In fact, most people return to their jobs right after the procedure. For more info on the National Spine & Pain Centers: *www.TreatingPain.com*

Smoking May Cause Disc Degeneration

As we age, the discs in our spine start to naturally break down due to everyday living. This is commonly known as disc degeneration, which can cause pain in the neck or back areas. This is felt by almost half of the population 40 years of age or older. When you reach 80 years old, sadly the rate doubles to a whopping 80%!

A 10-year study done at Mie University and Osaka University in Japan, and Rush University Medical Center in Chicago, Illinois have found that smokers tend to experience disc degeneration at greater rates than non-smokers. The study of 197 individuals over the age of 65 in Japan, revealed their disc height gradually reduced an average of 5.8% with nearly 55% experiencing degeneration in one or two of their discs. Other factors to avoid disc degeneration are maintaining a healthy diet, normal weight, and to avoid lifting heavy objects.

Plus, women are more vulnerable than men to disc degeneration. Researchers have found that chiropractic can help ease lower back pain, further reducing the likelihood that your discs will degenerate at a faster rate when you age. For more info see web: *www.ChiroNexus.net*

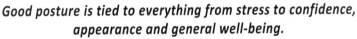

 Good posture is tied to everything from stress to confidence, appearance and general well-being.

Other Methods of Treatment

WATER THERAPY: has been used throughout history. Many ancient civilizations believed water – especially from hot mineral springs – had natural healing properties and they used it to treat various ailments, including muscle pain. This is known as Hydrotherapy. There is also a water therapy called Aquatic Therapy – essentially Physical Therapy conducted in the water – which is frequently used to manage various musculoskeletal conditions, including lower back pain. Warm or hot water transfers heat well, so being immersed in it causes blood vessels to dilate. This can decrease pain and allow increased mobility.

We have had painless bodies, and also have enjoyed natural hot mineral baths. They are soothing and relaxing to the body and mind and are a good preventive treatment!

CHIROPRACTIC / OSTEOPATHIC: involve physical and methodical repositioning of the head, shoulders, neck, back or hips to help alleviate any back pain by a Chiropractor or Osteopath respectively. It is noninvasive and does not require elaborate technology. The rate of serious complication from spinal manipulation appears to be very low overall. The most common side effects are sometimes minor discomfort in the treated area. Manipulation is not for everyone. It's not advised for people with back pain occurring with serious joint or bone disorders or a herniated disc.

TRACTION, CORSETS, BRACES AND BELTS: Some people experience pain relief when they are in traction, but it's usually short-lived. There is no evidence traction provides any long-term benefits for people with back pain. Although corsets, braces and belts may be appropriate for preventing injury, there is little evidence they help to treat low back pain. In fact, by preventing you from using your back and abdominal muscles, they may actually cause more problems than they solve by causing the muscles in your body's core to atrophy from under-use.

131

Expand your mind by learning something new.
Expand someone else's mind by sharing your knowledge.

Back Pain Treatments That Work
– From Dr. Joseph Mercola

"Worldwide, one in ten people suffer from lower back pain, and it's the #1 cause of job disability," according to fitness expert Dr. Joseph Mercola (*mercola.com*). "To avoid low-back pain which is the second most common symptom-related reason for doctor's visits in the U.S., here are some important tips to remember:

1. Stay Active. Most people want to 'baby' the pain and avoid moving, however a report in *The Guardian* found that exercise that strengthens the core, such as Yoga, Pilates and stretching, may be better than drugs and surgeries. Swimming may also be beneficial.

2. Stand up more. Simply standing up as much as possible each day may relieve back pain. When you sit for long periods of time you typically end up shortening your iliacus, psoas, and quadratus lumborum muscles that connect from your lumbar region to the top of your femur and pelvis. When these muscles are chronically short, it effectively pulls your lower back (lumbar) forward. Imbalance among the anterior and posterior chains of muscles leads to the pain you experience. By rebalancing and strengthening these muscles, you ease back pain. Also, when there's insufficient movement in your hip and thoracic spine, you end up with excessive movement in your lower back; the solution is to exercise regularly to keep your back and abdominal muscles strong and flexible (for more info on sitting too long see page 72).

3. Get a stand-up desk. It adjusts to suit your height and helps reduce back pain (page 72). Studies show that prolonged sitting may shorten your life, and standing up just 10-15 minutes per hour may make your back feel better."

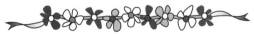

As a single footstep will not make a path on earth, so a single thought will not make a pathway in the mind. To make a deep physical path, we walk again and again. To make a deep spiritual path, we must think over and over the kind of thoughts we wish to dominate our lives. – Henry David Thoreau

Stress Reduction and Back Pain

Stress is a fact of life. We know if we are hyper-aware and hyper-responsive to the multitude of stressors we face daily, we start to "burn out" and become susceptible to a number of ailments, including depression and heart disease. On the musculoskeletal level, stress responses can cause muscles to tense in preparation for action, which can cause painful spasms. **Here are some techniques to help reduce daily stress:**

BREATHING EXERCISES: Try inhaling to count of three and exhaling to count of six. Repeat several times. (See *Bragg Super Power Breathing* book for more exercises.)

BODY SCAN: Begin by either lying or sitting down. Do the Breathing Exercise above. Once you feel relaxed, do a mental sweep of your body! Go slowly, noting areas of tightness or tension. Once you've finished the scan, return to those areas and let attention linger there. "Breathe into" those areas for several breathing cycles and imagine your muscles relaxing! This can help you become aware of the early warning signs of an impending back attack.

MEDITATION: Sit on a chair and observe your thoughts and emotions passing through you. Allow them to come and go without getting caught up in them, then watch them as they glide out of the room!

EXERCISE: Yoga, swimming, Tai chi and especially walking can help you reduce stress. More on walking see pages 57-61.

Your Posture and Back Pain

Bad posture can put excessive strain on certain portions of the spine, which may contribute to back problems. Proper posture aligns the head, chest and pelvis so that they are centered over one another with the body's weight centrally balanced (see more on posture pages 65-67). Stooped shoulders, slouching while sitting, or an excessive arch in the lower back can throw off the body's natural balance and put undue stress on certain muscles in the back, while leaving others under-used.

New Wearable Technology To Promote Posture

Functional apparel is available for those seeking pain relief with such products as AlignMed's patented *NeuroBand* technology which controls your posture to reduce back pain. They offer garments with built in or customizable elastic panels and bands used as controlled resistance to train the body to correct bad posture; reduce back pain; increase poise and confidence. *AlignMed.com*

Another device to aid in your posture is the *Lumo Lift*, a little sensor that you clip onto your shirt below your collarbone; it vibrates when you slouch. Patented biomechanic monitoring sensors in the *Lumo Lift* use angle displacement as a measure to let you know when your body slouches away from what you've calibrated as your standard of good posture.

Take Whiplash Injuries to Your Chiropractor

Chiropractic, in contrast to most treatments, has done well over the years helping prevent many whiplash injuries from becoming painful and chronic. Because of their high success record with treating whiplash injuries, researchers worldwide are studying chiropractic treatment methods. A group of medical researchers from Dublin, Ireland compared a treatment approach similar to that used by chiropractors with that of medication and rest. Sixty-one patients seen at the emergency room for whiplash injury were divided into two groups to receive these two different treatments. The group receiving chiropractic had the greater reduction of pain and return of movement than did the group treated with medication, rest and neck collars. These results led the researchers to conclude that whiplash is better treated with early active chiropractic treatment! Many people suffering from whiplash injury could avoid prolonged or permanent suffering by receiving chiropractic care. Physiotherapy and chiropractic should be used in treating whiplash. We have seen miracles and have benefitted ourselves when it was needed.

Chapter 14

Nature's Way to Healthy, Strong and Happy Feet

The basics of foot functions

Almost all of us are born with perfect feet. It's the abuse millions give their feet that makes them limp into adulthood crying, *"My aching feet are killing me!"*

The foot is a complex, elegant and delicately balanced miracle mechanism. Perfect balance is essential to foot comfort, and maintenance of this balance depends upon healthy natural foot function and a healthy body.

Almost all types of shoes made disturb the delicate balance of the feet. Some to the extent that the wearer cannot endure the jars and missteps in addition to walking on the hard city streets which can also upset the normal foot function. This results in either tension or locking of the joints, painful strain in the arches, muscles and limitation of foot motion or a combination of these disturbances. The direct consequence is a growing discomfort: aches and pains in the feet, legs, knees, thighs and back!

As long as your amazing, balanced foot function is maintained, your feet will be comfortable. No matter how out of shape your feet may appear, if they can be made to function at least 85% normally, then pain disappears, miracles happen and soon with loving care your feet will feel healthy again!

Now, let us demonstrate what we mean by foot function or the coordination of its many intricate parts. Do this experiment now – before you read further – and you will understand at once the natural or unnatural (as this may be) function of the feet. Stand on one foot (without shoes) and without support, try to maintain your balance for a few minutes. If your foot function is normal, balance will be maintained with perfect ease.

The foot, a work of art, is an engineering masterpiece!
– Leonardo da Vinci

Perfect Balance or No Balance

If foot function is impaired, balance will be difficult. You will tire in a short time and even sometimes in minutes can suffer leg pains. Observe what happens: at once the inner side of the foot comes into rapid play or action, with slight, constantly fluctuating adjustments necessary to sustain the body balance; the outer side of the foot remains comparatively immobile and your entire weight tends to focus upon that part.

The fluctuating inner part of the foot is called the *spring-arch*. Its chief function is to adjust for and maintain balance. The outer portion is called the *weight-bearing arch* and it operates to center and sustain the body weight.

By this simple experiment, you will learn not only the importance of the structure of your feet, but you will also be able to test their condition. The normal, unimpaired foot will balance the body perfectly, with graceful, easy movements and only a slight swaying of the body. The weak, crippled or deformed foot will make violent jerky efforts to balance the body, but will fail! Impaired function will force you to reach for support, to drop the other foot to the ground, or fall in a heap.

The condition of a great majority of feet are between the extremes of Perfect Balance and No Balance. The vital importance of this balancing action of the foot becomes evident the moment we consider the act of walking. While walking, we are continuously balancing first on one foot and then on the other as we transfer the weight of the body forward from right to left and left to right. In fact, it is a movement demanding remarkable equipoise, for the height and mass of the human body are out of proportion architecturally to the narrow base formed by the feet. The equilibrium, in turn, depends upon the perfect coordination of the nerves and muscles and their control of the lever-like bones, fulcrums, bases, angles and shifting surface of the feet. **Correct walking is a feat of balancing on balanced feet!**

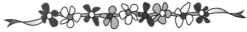

Women have four times as many foot problems as men do.

Since most all foot comfort depends upon normal foot function, beware of a diagnosis of arthritis or so-called rheumatism when the lower extremities are painful, since nearly all of these symptoms can stem from some functional foot disturbance to even being overweight and having poor posture. For more information refer to the section on gout (page 186), arthritis and rheumatism (pages 167-168).

Causes of Foot Problems

Nearly all foot troubles are the result of various injuries. The most common injury is caused by shoes that do not properly conform to the foot and hence, do not permit free and natural foot performance. Quite often, students are surprised when we tell them that their feet are not functioning normally. It is hard to make them understand that bones are actually dislocated. The reason this bone displacement occurs is simple and plausible. **The feet, relative to their size, do more work than any other part of the body! They are subjected to injury daily. Ill-fitting shoes, missteps, sprains, pounding on hard sidewalks, etc. all take their toll!** The cumulative effect of all of this punishment finally displaces the bones, upsets the balanced function and pain is the result. The body's *walking gear* is slowly being put out of adjustment!

Bad Walking Habits Bring Miseries

One of the early signs is the eversion, or outward turning of the foot. From here serious foot troubles start! This is walking out of natural foot and body balance and affects all of the foot bones and nerves, and in turn affects the ankle, calf, knee and hip! This can result in the knee being thrown out of balance, as well as the thighs. *The hip and lower spine are pushed out of alignment. The trouble travels up the spine, also resulting in misplacement of the shoulders and head. Pains and miseries are felt throughout the body.* This may be expected, when the feet are out of balance.

The human foot is often called the "mirror of your health."
Often feet provide an early indication of health conditions such as diabetes, arthritis and heart disease.

Again, let us say, these pains will be given many names from arthritis to curvature of the spine or you may be told you have slipped discs of the vertebrae, etc. The basic cause of all your pain, however, may be that you are completely out of foot-balance, thus throwing your entire body out of line!

The actual mechanism in the foot, after it becomes everted, is disturbed by a specific displacement of certain bones in the arches. These bones become jammed into a position of extreme tension that strains the ligaments and also the arch muscles. The results are a marked impairment of foot action and a complete change in weight-bearing forces. Due to changes in equilibrium, the body is thrown forward so that the muscles have to compensate and thus work overtime to keep the body erect. The body muscles are straining, just as if a person were continually walking downhill and holding the body erect to compensate for the grade. This effect brings into unnatural play the legs, back and neck muscles, which can soon become tired and ache!

 The fundamental abnormality, as it exists in the vast majority of cases, is a specific displacement of certain bones of the feet. This causes limited foot action and prolonged arch strain, these being two conditions which are usually responsible for disturbing foot pains.

Sadly – Foot Pain is Worldwide

It is very apparent foot pain is worldwide. In Australia, foot pain affects nearly 1 in 5 people. Problems include their balance and gait, and an increased risk of falls, impacting their overall health-related quality of life. The North West Adelaide Health Study of 4,060 people found those who were overweight or obese, had diabetes or cardiovascular disease, had a higher prevalence of foot pain. Females were 40% more likely to have pain than males, and people aged 50 years and over, were more likely to report foot pain. In the United Kingdom, a study of 3,417 people found 18% with joint pain in their feet, as well as swelling and stiffness. Those with chronic heel pain were 3 times more likely to be obese, and four times more likely to have flat feet.

The Many Causes of Foot Problems

- Shoes that mold and push the feet out of alignment cause mounting trouble unless shoes conform to the foot.

- Usage of unnatural and ill-fitting shoes, causing slow displacement of bones which limit foot and arch function and cause corns, bunions and foot problems.

- Women's high heels can cause a multitude of painful symptoms as a result of distorted foot functions, and also throw the body's posture and organs out of line.

- Deficiencies of proper nutrients and protein, which can prevent the building of a normal healthy foot.

- Deficiencies of the minerals like calcium and other bone-making nutrients can prevent the building and maintaining of healthy, strong feet.

- Insufficient and incorrect foot exercises, can result in weak feet. Foot muscles can't get full exercise when bound in shoes all the time (go barefoot more often).

- Bones of the feet require exercise to function correctly.

- All shoes hamper the full exercise of the 26 foot bones, also the ligaments don't get the exercise they need!

Be Aware of Cold Feet Problems

Cold feet could indicate poor circulation; peripheral vascular disease, poor blood supply or other possible systemic diseases such as diabetes or deep vein thrombosis. Foot problems such as gangrene are a result of poor blood supply. Cold feet could be the first sign of more serious foot problems which is why you should check with your physician immediately. Your doctor will generally assess skin temperature; skin color; your pulses in your feet, including dorsalis pedis and posterior tibial pulses. Another test may include the doppler ultrasound (preferable method).

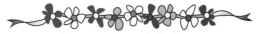

It's supposed to be a professional secret, but I'll tell you anyway. We doctors do nothing. We only help and encourage the doctor within.
– Albert Schweitzer, Philosopher & Physician

The Importance of Foot Education

We can plainly see that most foot troubles are mainly caused by ill-fitting shoes, lack of exercise, poor posture and various vitamin and mineral deficiencies. That is the reason this foot care program was written, to help you regain the feeling of healthy, strong, youthful feet!

No matter how deformed the feet may appear, if the nutrition and function can be improved, the pains will be lessened and the feet will feel stronger! To the health student this is very welcome news. It means that he or she may get comfort, even while having the worst-looking feet. But it also means that a person is not necessarily immune from functional and nutritional foot disorders simply because he or she possesses perfect-looking feet. Even beautiful looking feet may give you problems, too. What we really want are healthy, strong, serviceable feet that you can use for hours upon hours without the slightest sign of pain or fatigue! This is what we will strive for you in this *Foot Care Program*. No matter how much trouble you are experiencing with your feet, you are now going to treat them as Mother Nature intended you to and improvement will begin!!!

Go Barefoot for Healthy, Youthful Feet!

The first step in building healthy, new feet is to go barefoot at every opportunity, and please stop worrying about catching a cold when going barefoot (diabetics only go barefoot at home and it's best you wear socks). You don't catch colds from walking on cold floors or other surfaces. This old rumor should have been discarded hundreds of years ago! Colds are Mother Nature's way of purging the body of toxic poisons. They are the safety valve that lets the poisons leave the body. Think of all the body waste, mucus and poison released from your blood, nose and lungs, when you have a cold. **Remember the body has its own repair shop built right into it. Your miracle body when given the opportunity, is self-cleansing, self-repairing and self-healing!**

Be kind to each other – You can work miracles with kindness.
A little kindness can make a big difference! – Mother Teresa

Whenever you can get your shoes off (home, car, office, etc.), please do so! Most shoes, clogs, sandals and foot covers of all kinds can impede natural foot function. It's usually the combination of poor nutrition and improperly fitted shoes that cause most foot troubles, directly or indirectly.

Barefoot Promotes Happy, Healthy Feet

Although you can stretch out your toes, ankles and feet while wearing shoes, it is far more beneficial and relaxing to enjoy the ritual of stretching while barefoot!

By now, you may be aware of our philosophy of keeping your feet unhampered by shoes and socks as much as possible. Encourage friends and family to learn to enjoy going barefoot. Create a house rule that no one can wear shoes in your home! The Japanese have followed this practice for centuries. It is not only healthful, but you will find the carpets need to be vacuumed less frequently when shoes are removed upon entering the house.

If some friends seem a bit reluctant at first to go barefoot in your house, provide slippers for them. Keep a supply of inexpensive slippers at the front door. Before long, you will find that your friends will look forward to slipping off their shoes and they will probably bring along a pair of socks (tennis socks are ideal) or scuffs of their own when they visit. This is another way you can share your new-found knowledge about building strong, sturdy, healthy, happy feet!

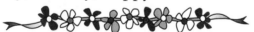

Shoes were unknown to our ancient forefathers; they went barefoot! But we squeeze our feet into shoes, losing direct contact with the ground. It's a central problem. It sounds trivial, but wearing shoes deprives our organs of the benefits provided by the reflex zones on our feet. What's worse is the lack of ventilation and constant pressure (caused by "fashionable" footwear that's often too tight and small) causing calluses, corns, hammertoes, and other deformities.
– Jurgen Jora, "Foot Reflexology A Visual Guide For Self-Treatment"

People who habitually go barefoot have stronger, healthier feet than those who wear shoes. – Society for Barefoot Living • BareFooters.org

Love is the sun shining in us to sparkle our lives and others! – Patricia Bragg

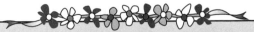

Benefits Of Walking Barefoot
5 Minutes Daily Are Astonishing

By walking barefoot we experience multiple benefits that we don't receive by walking with shoes. One of the more obvious benefits of walking barefoot is that we have a connection to the earth and it's magnetic field. Our body is conductive to the earth and the earth is conductive to our body. The earth is full of negative ions and we flood our body with negative ions by walking barefoot, this is also known as 'earthing' or grounding Earthing is the first and quite influential benefit of walking barefoot, but there are many other benefits of walking barefoot as well, such as:

1. Improving Sleep Quality: Walking barefoot relieves tension and removes positive ions to make way for negative ions. Negative ions are relaxing and help you improve sleep quality. Walking barefoot helps to balance your circadian rhythm to give you better awake/asleep conscious awareness.

2. Balance Electrons and Influence the Brain: Walking barefoot helps us to balance emotional and mental stability and spiritual well-being.

3. Develop and Increase Your Senses: When we remove our shoes we open up our senses and allow our nervous system to explore more.

4. Improves Your Overall Posture: When we begin to walk barefoot, run, jog and play with just our feet we can begin to strengthen our ankles, feet and toes again which gives us better balance, stability and posture.

India-China Foot Survey Proves Barefoot Best!

Perhaps nothing can illustrate the foregoing more graphically than a foot survey taken years ago in India and China among people who habitually go barefoot. In the United States, similar foot surveys and studies revealed that about 85% of the adult population is foot defective, whereas the India-China Survey of some 5,000 people showed only a low 7% incidence of foot defects! Please do take care of your foot health and protect your feet and total well-being! Never neglect your feet and health and become a burden to yourself and perhaps to your family and others! See web: *www.barefooters.org*

Researchers have discovered that the more healthy habits an individual practices, the longer they live and the healthier they are!
– Elizabeth Vierck, author, "Health Smart"

Written in the Pacific Paradise of Hawaii

We originally wrote this *Bragg Foot Care Program* at our home in Hawaii. The Hawaiian beach boys and girls, who seldom wear shoes, have perfect feet. In Hawaii, so many people go barefoot or wear just a light sandal that gives most Hawaiian's feet more freedom. As a result of going barefoot, these wonderful people of the Hawaiian Islands may just have the healthiest, happiest feet in the world. Almost everyone does the native Hula dance, which is never done in shoes or sandals of any kind!

We imagine what remark you might give us regarding this statement, "We cannot live in Hawaii and go barefoot and do the Hula dance." We thoroughly agree with you! But, we can learn a lesson from these happy people and go barefoot in our own homes and around our front and back yards. Even your local park lawn can be inviting! When we do wear shoes, they should be of the design that gives the bones and muscles as much flexible freedom as needed. When barefoot, your feet function more as wise Mother Nature intended.

Sick Feet Mar Beauty and Health

From this day forward, make it a practice to spend as much time as possible going barefoot. Let your feet live the Natural Way! Next to the heart, the feet carry the greatest work load of any body part. Keep this in mind when you backslide on your *Bragg Foot Care Program!*

Tired, aching feet and wearing badly-fitted shoes can make your face tense and your expression unhappy and contribute to backaches, bad posture and many other ills. What's more, you tend to drag such feet, and that ungraceful habit alone can make you feel and look years older than you are! Occasionally you may have a foot problem serious enough to require medical attention, but generally you can keep your feet in top shape all by yourself! It's not difficult to do and worth all the effort.

Many people go through life committing partial suicide – destroying their health, youth, energy and creativity. Indeed, to learn how to be good to oneself is often more difficult than to learn how to be good to others. – Joshua Liebman, Ph.D.

Bragg Foot Care Program

Here is your program for rejuvenating your feet and for bringing back the vitality, energy and spring in your step that belongs to them! Study this foot program seriously. Take the time to take care of your feet, then they will work hard and faithfully for you if you will give them the care and attention they need and deserve!

Your Feet Actually Work Best Without Shoes

Research by physical therapist, Michael Warburton of Australia, found that running barefoot decreases the likelihood of ankle sprains, plantar fasciitis and chronic injuries (*mercola.com*). Warburton revealed that wearing footwear actually increases the chances of getting an ankle sprain, one of the most common sports injuries, because it either decreases your awareness of foot position or increases the twisting torque on your ankle, especially during a stumble. Your feet were designed to work best without shoes. When you surround your feet with extra padding like athletic shoes, your foot muscles are not being used appropriately. There are obviously some concerns with going barefoot, namely stepping on a sharp object or rock and injuring your skin. But if done properly, walking and even running barefoot can be quite safe.

Your Natural Gait When Barefoot is Best

A "fox gait" or fox-walking, is the graceful flow of your body in total synchronization when you walk barefoot. Your knees are bent, rather than locked, the ball of your foot touches the ground first, followed by your heel; this is your natural gait. In contrast, a "cow-walk" puts tremendous pressure on your joints, starting with squeezing your foot inside a shoe, jarring the knees as they are locked straight upon the pole-driving impact of the heel, which then travels straight up your spine, all the way up to your neck. Your feet no longer naturally adjust to your gait for optimum efficiency and safety, because of wearing shoes.

Prevention is always preferable to the cure.

Earthing: Walking and Living Barefoot

Historically, humans have lived a barefoot lifestyle where they walked, slept, and lived in complete contact with Mother Earth. If worn, shoes were made of animal skins, which gave direct contact to the Earth. When observing modern day humanity, notice that few people go barefoot anymore. The human body acts as a conductive device when our bare feet come into contact with the Earth and give us a charge of energy which helps to restore a natural electrical balance in our body.

There are many ways to restore this natural balance, commonly known as *Earthing* or *Grounding*. The basis of Earthing is to connect our bodies with the Earth, by walking barefoot on grass, sand, and dirt, and by sleeping on grounded sheets if unable to sleep on the ground. Earthing allows the Earth's surface, which is abundant in negative-charged, free electrons, to interact with our bodies and act as a giant anti-inflammatory agent. In one study on the effects of Grounding and secretion of cortisol (known as the *stress hormone*), Dr. Maurice Ghaly, retired anesthesiologist, determined that Earthing during sleep "resynchronizes cortisol secretion in alignment with its natural, normal rhythm." To that effect, the people in the study reported that they experienced better sleep and less pain.

One may ask: how can I reap the benefits of Earthing? First and most important, we must go barefoot outdoors as often as possible! Walking barefoot on grass, sand, or dirt all allow our bodies to absorb these electrical charges from the Earth's surfaces. For those unable to do so, it's advised to buy a grounded floor mat for your bare feet to use under your office desk, or in your home area. Go barefoot whenever possible! Go outside and stroll barefoot, or enjoy a nap lying on your healthy home grass.

For more info on "Earthing" check out these webs:

- *www.Earthing.com* • *www.EarthingInstitute.net*
- *www.Mercola.com* • *www.DoctorOz.com*

Foot Problems – Common at Any Age

Even youth can have foot pain. Heel pain is common in very active children ages 8-13, when high-impact exercises and physical activity can irritate growth centers of the heel.

Pregnant women tend to have special foot problems from weight gain, swelling in their feet and ankles and the release of hormones that cause ligaments to relax. These hormones help women bear their child, but can weaken the feet. Raised hormone levels can cause water retention during pregnancy, making pregnant women swollen and bloated.

At work, an estimated 120,000 job-related foot injuries occur every year, about a third of them involving the toes. Other feet problems include the pinched nerves between the toes; plantar fasciitis and tarsal tunnel syndrome.

Restore Ideal Neutral Position of the Feet

The foot is made up of 26 bones and 33 joints, layered with 120 muscles, ligaments and nerves. Most people take about 3,000 to 4,000 steps per day, each placing a force of 2 to 3 times their body weight on the feet!

A solution to foot pain can be found in orthotic insoles, often these provide low-cost, long-lasting relief. They help restore ideal neutral position of the feet and help correct over-pronation, see: *TheInsoleStore.com.*

Tea Tree Oil for Athlete's Foot, Fungus & Smelly Feet

Apply tea tree oil lightly right from the bottle on affected areas. Full strength may over-dry the skin. If this happens dilute oil by mixing 1/3 tea tree oil with 2/3 olive oil or Jojoba oil. Apply to the area three times a day. Continue treatment for one week after the problem disappears.

For smelly feet, you can enjoy a tea tree oil foot soak. Add 5-10 drops to warm water in a shallow pan. Do nightly and continue until you experience improvement.

The oil derived from tea tree leaves can be used for treating skin abrasions, acne, canker sores and foot fungus, says William Keller, Ph.D., Herbal expert and Chair of Dept. of Pharmaceutical Sciences at Samford University.

Chapter 15

Give Proper Loving Care To Your Feet That Carry You Through Life!

Clean feet are important

Like the rest of your body, feet perspire. Each foot has thousands of sweat glands and because they're usually encased in shoes, socks or stockings, they retain more perspiration than less-restricted parts of the body. This can lead to unpleasant odors and accumulation of rough or dead skin that cause irritation and soreness.

You must tackle foot-bathing with real dedication and vigor. Keep the following items handy, right next to your tub or shower: a hand brush with moderately stiff bristles, a worn-out toothbrush and a pumice stone.

Now first, scrub your feet with the hand brush. Use health soaps (*tea tree, vegetable, herbal, oatmeal or glycerine*) and warm water. Do not neglect the soles of the feet. Next, gently scrub between the toes. Here's where you use the toothbrush, because these places are hard to get at otherwise. It's particularly important to get your feet absolutely clean because this helps to prevent athlete's foot, which is one of the most irritating of foot problems.

(147)

Now rinse feet and while they're still wet, (if in shower sit down on handy shower stool) rub pumice stone or foot file lightly on foot parts that feel rough. This usually includes the heels and balls of feet. Use the stone with a gentle, rotary motion, as this helps to soften the skin and discourages heavy calluses from forming.

The average American has their feet encased in shoes for over 12 hours daily and most often the shoes are ill-fitting, resulting in foot problems.

I cannot think clearly when my feet hurt!
– President Abraham Lincoln, 16th US President

If you pick them up, O' Lord, I'll put 'em down. – Prayer of Tired Walker

Drying your feet is very important! Athlete's foot is caused by a fungus that thrives on warm, damp skin. If you do not dry the feet thoroughly, especially between the toes, you are inviting this fungus which is difficult to overcome. Do not scrub-dry the areas between your toes. Pat them dry, gently but firmly, otherwise, you may irritate these areas. The rest of the foot you may dry vigorously. In fact, this form of brief massage has the added advantage of stimulating foot circulation.

Pedicure and Trimming The Toenails

A good time to give yourself a pedicure is after your foot bath, when skin is warm and moist. You can gently push back the cuticle and rid toenails of excess cuticle that forms around the nails. This habit prevents cuticles from growing wild. *(If you choose salon pedicures be sure that the foot tub is cleaned and the instruments are sterilized or take your own.)*

When trimming your toenails, please never rip any off. This may leave a ragged torn edge that can become extremely sensitive to shoe pressure. Also, never trim down into the corners of a nail as this is one of the chief causes of ingrown toenails. Trim toenails straight across and leave the corners alone. Ingrown toenails, corns, calluses, bunions and Athlete's Foot – all detract from the health, appearance and happiness of your feet!

Remember that the basic purpose of foot hygiene is to maintain a healthy tone and vigor in each foot, just as strengthening-up exercises are designed to keep the body trim! Hygienic foot-care is a routine habit that pays great dividends in healthier feet to carry you through life.

Finish off your pedicure with a massage using olive oil to keep your feet flexible, soft and smooth. This oil is also great for the legs, arms, face and entire body.

Every man is the builder of a temple called his body. We are all our own sculptors and painters and our material is our own flesh, blood and bones. – Henry David Thoreau, American author and poet

Relaxation techniques are very important benefits to the body's general health and cardiovascular system. Such techniques as sitting quietly, deep breathing, meditation and ignoring distracting thoughts can bring down blood pressure and are free of side effects. – Harvard Health Letter

Inspect Your Feet to Keep them Healthy

Perform a foot self-exam once a week when you take a bath or shower. As you are drying off your feet, take a good look on the soles for any scaling and between your toes for any peeling areas. These spots could signal the presence of athlete's foot. Also look for discoloration of the nails, which could indicate a nail fungus. If you have diabetes, you should inspect your feet every day since diabetes can lead to a higher risk of foot sores and infections. Don't attempt to self-treat painful foot woes. Any pain, redness, swelling, or discoloration that persists should be checked out by a podiatric physician. Protect your feet in public areas. Be sure to wear shower shoes at the gym, in locker rooms, and at public pools. These places tend to be breeding grounds for fungi that can lead to infections.

Foot Bath and Foot Massage

The following special foot bath will prove beneficial. Sit on a chair next to the bathtub with your feet dangling under the tap. Turn on the tap to make a strong flow for 5 to 10 minutes, alternating hot and cold water over your feet (diabetic and heart patients please use caution when using hot water). If you have a spray attachment, just spray alternating directly hot, then cold water, on your feet – it feels so great!

After this special foot bath, dry your feet thoroughly with a rough towel and be sure that all the moisture is off your feet. Now sprinkle cornstarch over your feet and start your foot massage, using fingers, mainly thumbs, in a circular motion. Start on the bottoms of the feet. Put plenty of cornstarch on your hands and massage the soles of your feet in rotary motion. With both hands, twist each foot back and forth in opposite directions to keep them limber and healthy. Then massage the sides and ankles in a rotary motion. Also, gently pull and twist each toe from its base. End up with a stroking massage motion. Don't be afraid to use pressure as this promotes more healthy blood circulation to the general structure of the feet and ankles, and helps push the toxins and crystals out of the feet!

Please keep in mind that massage is very important in making your feet healthy, happy and tingling with vitality. Circulation reaches its weakest point in the feet because the heart has to drive blood there. They are farthest from the heart and blood must flow against gravity to return to the heart. Hence, circulation may become sluggish in the feet (cold and aching feet are two of the signs of poor circulation). See page 221 for more info on foot reflexology, a specialized and very pleasant, relaxing, powerful healing technique to enjoy.

Baby Your Tired, Aching Feet

Tired, hurting feet can take the joy out of your life! This book is filled with ways to bring life back to your feet! Some methods are a little more elaborate than others, but all are just variations of foot care therapy: various special foot soaks (herbal, vinegar, Epsom salts), foot therapy, pedicure, massage, exercise and rest.

Tips To Do Away with Smelly Feet:

Your feet have about half a million sweat glands, and when you wear socks and shoes, the sweat gets trapped inside. Bacteria and fungus can thrive in this type of warm, moist environment, and can produce odor. **Another good reason to go barefoot!** To truly eliminate the aroma you need to deal with both your feet and your socks and shoes. Here's how:

- **Apple cider vinegar baths:** For clean smelling feet – soak your feet daily in one part vinegar and two parts water. The aim is to reduce the level of bacteria that causes odor.

- **Purchase good socks and shoes:** To prevent stinky feet from starting in the first place, purchase socks and shoes made of breathable materials. Synthetic materials provide less ventilation than natural materials, and so polyester or nylon socks may increase the amount of perspiration compared to cotton. Natural materials (such as cotton or wool) generally provide more ventilation and therefore may limit the growth of bacteria.

- **Never, ever go sock-less:** Wearing shoes without socks can lead to sweat accumulation, enabling bacteria to grow over time. Also, there can be dead skin cells, dirt, oils, and fungus thriving in there.

- **Wash socks and rotate shoes:** Socks should be changed every day to prevent the buildup of moisture and dead skin – sometimes more than once, if you're particularly sweaty or it's really hot out. Air out your shoes 24-hours between wearings.

Remember the longest journey starts with just one step.

Chapter 16

Exercises For Your Feet

The importance of exercise

If we are to be free from foot injuries of all kinds, regardless of our age, we must keep them strong and sturdy with exercises! The muscles, bones and tendons all need vigorous exercise to give them the great power to withstand the strain we put upon them. A regular foot program should be followed daily, with sufficient time and attention devoted to your precious, priceless feet.

There's one fact universally overlooked, feet are encased in shoes for about 12 hours a day. In this time, their activity is limited and the full freedom for normal exercising of the tissues, muscles and tendons is inhibited! During the remaining hours, the feet are inactive or in bed asleep. *(For foot comfort use a pillow to elevate blankets off of your feet to prevent drop foot problems.)* For almost the full 24 hours, the feet get little exercise, fresh air, sunshine (vitamin D3) and remember your feet need freedom time (no shoes). This lack of activity offers a sharp contrast to the vigorous and constant foot-movements of shoeless natives in tropical warm climates (many are world racing/running champs).

Treatments for tired feet are all very well, but obviously it would be far better to avoid tired feet altogether. You can help in this respect with exercises to strengthen your feet. The stronger and more supple your feet are (with increased blood circulation activity), the less apt you will be to collapse your body at the end of a hard day.

Exercises for Healthy Feet and Toes

Here are some easy-to-do foot strengtheners. Learn what they are designed to do and how they are done. Do these exercises in your bare feet, with absolutely no foot coverings, not even thin hosiery on your feet.

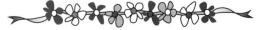

Make your two feet your best friends. – J. M. Barrie

Healthy Foot and Toe Exercises

Exercise No. 1: Stand with your feet parallel, toes straight ahead, rise up on your toes, then slowly come down. Do this about 20 times. This is the best warm-up exercise for the muscles and tendons of your feet.

Exercise No. 2: While seated, with your shoes and hosiery off, try picking up children's marbles, or something similar, with your toes. Don't use the same set of toes each time. Pick up the marbles with toes of one foot, let them drop to the floor, then try it with the toes of the other foot. Do this for 5 minutes daily. It's fun. At first, you may find it difficult to grasp the marbles with your toes, but after a few tries it becomes easier! All of the long tendons attached to the toes are strengthened by this exercise, and toes acquire more power to grip the ground and balance the feet.

Exercise No. 3: Stand barefoot on a thick, wide book so that the toes overlap the edge of the book. Move the toes over the edge of the book and grip. This should be done for several minutes each day. With each successive day the toes will show increased agility, and they will eventually be able to bend straight down, while the rest of the foot is horizontal. This strengthens the important toe tendons.

Exercise No. 4: While seated, place a pencil between your toes and try to write a letter. If this exercise is practiced for awhile, a legible letter may eventually be written. This uses the whole muscular structure of the foot, as well as the toes.

Exercise No. 5: While seated, firmly hold your foot with one hand. With your other hand, take your big toe and rotate it around firmly, first one direction and then the other, then gently pull each toe. Now repeat this exercise on all toes. This keeps toes limber and helps reduce any (big toe) bunions.

Little things are like weeds – the longer we neglect them, the larger they grow! – Croft M. Pentz, author of Christian books

---

It's strange that some men will drink and eat anything put before them, but will check very carefully the oil they put in their car.

Rolling Pin Foot Exercises

These are great exercises for the feet. Use a rolling pin, either plain or a model specifically designed for foot therapy (with knobs). The latter is wonderful for reaching the reflex points of the feet. Keep the rolling pin in your living room so it will always be handy to use when you are watching TV.

Exercise No. 1: While seated, roll the pin from the toes to the heel, putting all the pressure you can take on the entire soles on both the right foot and the left foot at the same time.

Exercise No. 2: Now stand and roll the pin from toes to heel, putting all the pressure you can first with one foot, then the other. This is an excellent exercise for building new feet from old. Every muscle, every bone, every nerve and tendon of the foot is ironed into its proper place. Spend plenty of time rolling the pin under the arches. You will feel the tiny crystals that may have formed, but with regular foot exercises, massage, reflexology and proper nutrition, these may soon disappear. These rolling pin exercises will pay you great dividends in foot health.

Vigorous Foot Walking Exercises

After a workout on the feet with the rolling pin, you are now ready to give the foot muscles, bones, nerves and tendons a workout for 10 minute sessions.

- Walk around on the **outer edges** of the feet.
- Walk around on the **inner edges** of the feet.
- Walk around just on **your heels.**
- Walk around just on **tiptoes.**

Walking this way may seem awkward, but these exercises will help strengthen and improve your feet.

Brisk walking performs physical, mental and spiritual miracles and wards off diseases, reduces stress and improves heart health, circulation, helps normalize weight, blood pressure and cholesterol.
– PBS T.V. Mark Fenton, author "Pedometer Walking: Stepping Your Way to Health, Weight Loss and Fitness"

Trust yourself – be wise, then you will know how to live.
– Johann Wolfgang von Goethe

Enjoy Barefoot Ground Contact Exercises

When possible walk barefoot on your grass or park lawns as often as possible. *Caution: call and check to avoid parks and golf course lawns if toxic chemicals are used!*

If you can walk on a sandy beach you are giving the feet the greatest of all tonics! When you walk on the beach your feet are walking naturally. Every part of the foot is activated as it should be. We have seen people with the most crippled and battered feet spend several months or more at a beach and emerge with whole new feet! Whether it be in Florida, California, Hawaii, or any other sandy spot, walking on the sand will do as much for your heart and soul as it will for your feet. With its uneven, undulating surface and deep drifts that become smooth at the water's edge, the beach is an ideal place to walk giving your entire foot a massage with each step!

Learn Lessons from Wise Mother Nature

Walking on the lawn or sand is the finest of all foot exercises! It acts as a stimulant to all the foot tissues. A child's ordinary sandbox or even smooth, small "pea" gravel in a box is ideal for this exercise. The sand or gravel fits the contours of the sole and the arch, acting as a healthy foot and ankle stimulator at the same time.

The most significant points to remember about foot exercising are: (1) at least one-half hour daily must be devoted to foot improvement, and (2) the exercises must be followed with faithful regularity. Only under these conditions, plus your healthy nutritional diet and foot therapy schedule, will any gratifying results be realized!

Your Dynamic Foot 'Springiness' Plan

No matter how you have abused your feet in the past, the foot program will help you! Carry a picture in your mind of the kind of feet you wish to mold through this foot care program. Let nothing stop you as you work on your schedule for attaining healthier, stronger feet that are going to carry you through your entire long life!

When recovering from accidents or fractures, it is best to take extra natural, mineral and vitamin supplements to nourish and help your body heal faster.

Chapter 17

Foot Care Through Life

Check your overall lifestyle and habits

When you find yourself in need of treatment, there are a number of factors you must consider before embarking upon a particular course. Your overall lifestyle is one of the first things on the list. In most cases your diet, sleeping habits, physical and mental activities, hobbies, occupation and geographical climate will play a part in your general health or lack thereof. Be sure to examine your mental, emotional and spiritual state of being as well. Know yourself! An honest appraisal of these factors will yield valuable information that will be very useful in determining the best way to treat any of your problems so you can plan, plot and take action to make yourself healthy!

Please keep in mind that foot diseases and conditions, especially chronic ones, are just like any other type of malady in that they are usually a direct result of certain actions, activities and lifestyles. Because of this, some people will be more likely to develop specific foot problems than others. For example, people whose jobs require them to be on their feet all day, like teachers, clerks, dentists, doctors, nurses, and athletes, are more inclined to develop recurrent foot problems than people in more sedentary careers.

Foot Care During Pregnancy

Because of weight gain and postural changes during pregnancy, foot and leg fatigue can become pronounced. There may be tiredness and heaviness, leg cramping and even the development of varicose veins. In most cases, these symptoms will disappear after the baby is born. In any case, proper foot care during pregnancy is important for the health of both mother and child.

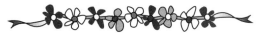

Babies and giving birth are blessings and miracles of life.
– Patricia Bragg, Pioneer Health Crusader

Wearing comfortable shoes to support you is vital. These should have the lowest and broadest heel that feels good. Since your feet might swell, especially in hot weather, the shoe must be large and flexible enough to allow for changes in foot size. There should be no hard pressure on the top of the foot or on the toes.

Don't wear shoes made of plastic, patent leather or synthetics that aren't flexible, and *will not give* with your foot. Your shoes should allow your feet to be flexible and breathe. The soles and heels are especially important. They should provide adequate support and cushioning without jarring or binding you. Flexible rubber or crepe soles, which are firm, yet springy, are generally better than hard leather bottoms. Women are best to avoid high heels, since pregnancy already changes your posture, why do further damage by misaligning yourself?

Your socks and stockings should be large enough to allow free toe movement. If you are advised to wear *support* hosiery, don't wear the tight advertised elastic hose – as it causes undue compression of the feet and legs. Instead, buy toeless (and sometimes heelless) seamless surgical hosiery and you can wear your usual hose or socks over them. Be careful that your socks do not have tight elastic bands which interfere with blood flow and can increase swelling.

The Relationship Between Estrogen & Collagen

According to a study at the University of Iowa, hormones could be the real culprit behind the majority of female foot pain. They found that pregnancy can lead to permanent foot changes that increase the risk for foot problems, while menopause can make a woman's feet more vulnerable to pain and injury. Dr. Michael Nirenberg, a podiatric physician, explains, *"When hormone levels drop during menopause, it causes a decrease in the production of collagen – a matrix of elastic tissue that's crucial for keeping the feet's supporting structures strong."* To help keep your feet strong and healthy do the *Bragg Foot Exercises* for the best results!

A strong, healthy body makes a strong, healthy mind.
– Thomas Jefferson, 3rd U.S. President, 1801-1809

Elevate, Exercise and Rest Your Feet

Raising and resting your feet on a pillow at night for sleeping, during a noon nap or when watching TV in the evening can help cut down swelling and cramping. While your feet are elevated, try flexing them, gripping with your toes, then curling them back, rotating your feet both ways at the ankles, and any other movements which increase your circulation and ease of motion. Follow the *Bragg Foot Care Program,* do the foot and walking exercises and faithfully follow The Bragg Health Lifestyle and healthy diet, plus go barefoot whenever possible. Mother – give yourself and your baby the best possible first steps into their new healthy life!

Caring for Children's Feet from Birth

When the fetus is only six weeks old, the feet and legs have already begun to develop. At birth, the average infant's foot length is slightly a little over three inches. Eventually, the feet will grow to about 8 inches (average) in length for women, and about 11 inches in length for a man. To promote proper foot development, the baby's feet should be monitored and attended to carefully.

157

Barefoot is Best, Especially for Babies!

The bones in their little feet are still soft and not yet fully formed. Why compress them with shoes? Give their bare feet a chance to move, wiggle, stretch and grow without any restriction. Don't constrict circulation and motion of the baby's developing, growing feet with *prison-like* shoes!

The only reason to cover your infant's feet is to keep them warm. To do so, use non-stretch socks of natural fabric, or a onesie baby garment with feet and legs, as long as the garment is not too tight. Check for shrinkage after washing and be sure your baby hasn't outgrown it. When covering the infant with a blanket, don't tuck it in too tightly. Either tuck loosely or allow the blanket to simply rest on the feet and legs. Free movement is the key.

Love begins by taking care of the loved ones at home. – Mother Teresa

Your Baby Needs Love and Massages

Your baby's position in the crib is also important. Don't let your baby always lie on their stomach. Turn the baby at intervals while sleeping. This helps promote balanced muscular development and prevents problems such as toenails which are curved in toward the toes due to a constant on-the-belly resting position. When diapering your child, notice whether the feet, legs, and bottom are symmetrical. If you see any difference between the two sides, consult your doctor. Also, do not diaper baby with bulky diapers. These force the legs into an unnatural, outward position causing bow legs. Fortunately now, most diaper materials are thin enough to prevent this problem. Before or after diapering, gently massage your baby's feet, spine, and entire body when time allows to promote nerve development and healthy circulation. **Remember foot and body massages are good for all ages!**

Do not dangle your baby from their arms to get him or her to walk faster. This puts strain on the arms, neck, spine and entire system. Respect Mother Nature's timetable; your child will stand and walk only when the foot and leg muscles are ready to support and move the entire body. Generally, an infant will attempt to crawl at about six months, try to stand at eight, will be able to stand well at about 12 months, and will walk unaided at 14 months or more. These are averages and have nothing to do with your child's ultimate coordination, as each child develops at its own rate.

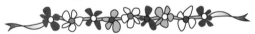

The U.S. Congress should immediately ban all ads aimed at children that promote foods high in fat and sugar – these unhealthy, nutrient-poor, high-calorie foods become life-long eating habits that are potentially life-threatening! The fast foods industry and their thousands of restaurants serve millions of meals daily that accelerate the growth of fast foods and have changed America's eating habits! Obesity is now an epidemic!
– Marion Nestle, Ph.D., M.P.H., author, "Food Politics, How the Food Industry Influences Nutrition and Health"

May you live healthy all the days of your life. – Jonathan Swift, writer

The Feet of Youth

It has been estimated that one-third of young children in this country have abnormal foot posture. This means that one out of every three people growing up in America is presently headed for aches, pains and worse throughout the years due to the fact that no one took the time or trouble to examine, care for and if necessary, correct the youth's foot problems.

It is true that almost all of us are born with perfect feet and that, naturally, the foot will develop well. But parents must examine their children's feet and encourage proper foot care habits in order to give them a good start on the path of healthy feet for life!

When your youngster begins to get up on his or her feet in the playpen, put a blanket or soft rug over the bottom pad. This will allow your child to begin to grip with the toes and to stand on a soft, yet firm surface. When he or she begins to walk, don't worry about awkwardness of movement or the lack of an arch on the foot. Unless a baby is exceptionally thin, there is a fatty pad under the arch which won't disappear until two-and-a-half or three years of age, and then the foot arch starts to show.

159

Some Simple Tips for Children's Foot Health

Many adult foot problems can start in childhood. That is why it is necessary to see that your child's feet are properly cared for. Neglecting foot health when young can lead to leg and back problems later in life. Children's feet grow very fast and by 12-16 months their feet have reached almost half adult size. This is a critical time to pay attention to foot health. Children can suffer from some of the same foot problems as adults.

Remember, foot health begins in childhood and that the child's feet must carry them for a lifetime. Their life is certain to be happier if you help them develop strong, healthy feet as they grows to maturity.

Here are some wise tips and hints to keep in mind:

- Replace shoes with a larger size as soon as necessary.
- Teach children to go toe straight ahead when walking. Toeing out or toeing in weakens the feet and throws the entire body out of alignment.
- When fitting stockings, allow ¼ longer than the longest toe (in a standing position).
- Bathe children's feet at least 2-3 times a week in lukewarm water and mild soap.
- Cut toe nails straight across and as long as the toe. Do not round corners – could cause ingrown toenails.
- Keep children's shoes in good repair.
- Provide a healthy nourishing balanced diet.

Monitor Children's Feet and Their Walking and Choose Children's Shoes Wisely

Unfortunately, one can't walk around the modern world barefoot forever! When it comes time to fit your child with shoes, use the same guidelines that you use to select your own comfortable shoes.

It's important to consistently inspect the way your child walks when he begins to do so. The best time to examine your child's gait is when he is barefoot, not when wearing tight, non flexible shoes! Does the child toe in or toe out consistently? Is he or she knock kneed or bow legged to an unusual degree? Does your youngster limp consistently, or walk only on the toes or heels?

None of these conditions are necessarily cause for alarm, but all should be checked by a pediatrician, orthopedist or podiatrist and also a chiropractor! The condition may be transient and hopefully disappear by itself with proper posture and guidance. However, it may be caused by improper bone or muscle development, perhaps due to faulty nutrition or defective metabolic functioning, etc. Check with an expert, it is the only way to be sure!

Have you ever looked at a newborn's foot? They are pudgy and relatively flat. All toddlers under 16 month have flat feet. Their arches don't fully develop until they reach 7-8 years of age.
– Stephanie Tourles, author, "Natural Foot Care"

As you bathe and massage your child, examine their feet. Look especially for small growths. A corn, callus or wart may be an indication of an underlying condition which is correctable if caught early! Inspect the nails, some develop a nail-biting problem. If the area around the nails is tender due to tearing or biting, soak the feet in warm water and add 1 Tbsp. apple cider vinegar. Also wrapping the foot for 10 to 15 minutes can help relieve pain and hasten healing. If nail-biting is severe, promptly consult your pediatrician.

Growing pains – the cramps in the legs some children get between 2 and 5 years old are no longer considered normal. There is a reason: poor posture, fatigue or faulty nutrition. Relief can be given by multiple vitamin and mineral supplements (especially calcium, magnesium and vitamin D), massaging, keeping the bedroom temperature warm enough, and by making sure one leg doesn't continually rest on the other during sleep. If growing pains persist, please see your health practitioner.

Children's Shoes Should Fit Right & Be Flexible

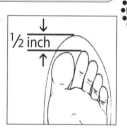

Children's shoes should be fitted so that when the child is standing, the shoe toe box is at least a half-inch longer than the longest toe (not necessarily the big toe). The shoe should not press down on the child's toes or on top of foot. The shoe should fit snugly, but not tightly at the heel. The heel should be firmly cradled and not slip or wiggle in the shoe as this can cause painful blisters.

The shoe itself should be flexible, with a shock-absorbing sole and heel, and should allow the foot to breathe. Shoes which come high on the ankles are not necessary. Ankles must be allowed to strengthen so as to support the body weight and to develop flexibility. Under no circumstances should you cram your child's feet into stylish, grown-up shoes or boots such as miniature high heels or cowboy boots. It's best to keep the shoe light, roomy and the sole flexible!

A healthy body, bones and feet come from healthy foods, habits and lifestyle. – Patricia Bragg, Health Crusader

By the same token, do not buy shoes that are far too large for your youngster's foot on the theory that he or she will grow into them. How would you like to have to walk around in shoes two sizes too large and get blisters and calluses because your feet will someday enlarge with age? Buy your child shoes that fit correctly, right now! Beware of hand-me-downs and resoled shoes that don't fit well. If any foot or walking problem arises, see a foot doctor to get at the cause of the difficulty; don't just cover it up or try to force the foot to change.

When your child has worn his or her new shoes for a day or two, check the feet for signs of any irritations. Sometimes these can be avoided by working the shoe at a particular spot, or by changing or loosening the lacing pattern. If the irritation persists, change the shoes. Proper footwear does not require much breaking in, since it is often the foot that is being broken! Socks, too, should be checked to ensure that they are not too small, haven't shrunk in the wash and do not bind the foot or restrict circulation. Remember, getting your child off on a good footing will pay dividends in ease, comfort and freedom of movement throughout their long, healthy, happy life!

Senior Foot Steps

Years of wear and tear can be hard on our feet. So can poor circulation, improperly trimmed toenails, and wearing shoes that don't fit properly. Problems with our feet can be the first sign of serious medical conditions such as arthritis, diabetes, nerve and circulatory disorders.

Practice good foot care daily. Check your feet regularly, or have a member of your family check them. It also helps to keep blood circulating to your feet as much as possible. Put your feet up. Try to avoid pressure from shoes that don't fit right. Try not to expose your feet to cold temperatures. Don't sit for long periods of time (especially with legs crossed, see page 71). Please don't smoke.

He who has health has hope; and he who has hope, has everything.
– Arabian proverb

As we age, changes in the feet happen naturally. Older feet tend to spread and change shape slightly. You might find your shoes, as a senior, increase by one size to accommodate the gradual spreading. This is normal, as is the reduction in the amount of fatty padding of the soles. The skin often dries and thins on older feet, resulting in cracking and inflammation. This can be reduced or eliminated by using olive oil and moistening creams and following this *Bragg Foot Care Program.*

With age, blood supply to the feet often diminishes, causing cold feet, fatigue and sometimes numbness. Moderate exercise helps alleviate this common problem.

Arthritis, another common difficulty of ageing, may be felt especially in the feet. Basically, arthritis is a condition affecting various joints. There may be a decrease or increase in space between bones, a breakdown of part of a bone, or a growth of bony bumps.

Investing in good, proper fitting shoes will help keep your feet healthy and happy and will add to your overall feeling of well-being. Remember, your feet carry you through life – so be extra loving and caring to them!

As a senior, you have a responsibility to yourself to keep your feet healthy so that as you age, you can still participate in and enjoy life's daily activities.

Prove to Yourself You Can Have Healthy Feet

Day by day, by faithfully following this natural *Bragg Foot Care Program,* you will see wonderful changes in your feet. They will be supple, flexible and free from pain. You will regain the feeling of springiness in your new feet. Is this worth working for? Just how important are your feet to you? Remember they must carry you through life! So you should treat them with your full faithful respect, so they can be healthy, happy feet and your constant pain-free companions with every step you take!

Self discipline is your golden key; without it, you can't be happy and healthy. – Maxwell Maltz, M.D., author

Good health and good sense are two of life's greatest blessings. – Publilius Syrus, Latin writer, 42 B.C.

Exercise and Eat for Total Health

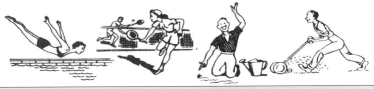

Enjoy Bragg Healthy Lifestyle
For a Lifetime of Super Health

In a broad sense, The Bragg Healthy Lifestyle for the Total Person is a combination of physical, mental, emotional, social and spiritual components. The ability of the individual to function effectively in his environment depends on how smoothly these components function as a whole. Of all the qualities that comprise an integrated personality, a totally healthy, fit body is one of the most desirable . . . so start today to achieve your health goals!

A person may be said to be totally physically fit if he functions as a total personality with efficiency and without pain or discomfort of any kind. This is to have a painless, tireless, ageless body. One possessing sufficient muscular strength and endurance to maintain a healthy posture and successfully carry on the duties imposed by life and the environment. To be able to handle emergencies and have enough energy for recreation and social obligations after the "work day" has ended. It is to meet the requirements of his environment through possessing the resilience to recover rapidly from fatigue, tension, stress and strain of daily living without the aid of stimulants, drugs or alcohol. To be able to enjoy natural recharging sleep at night and awaken fit and alert in the morning for the challenges of the new fresh day ahead.

Keeping the body totally healthy and fit is not a job for the uninformed or the careless person. It requires an understanding of the body and of a healthy lifestyle and then following it for a long, happy lifetime of health! The result of "The Bragg Healthy Lifestyle" is to wake up the possibilities within you, rejuvenate your body, mind and soul to total balanced health. It's within your reach, so don't procrastinate, start today! Our hearts and prayers go out to touch you with nourishing, caring love for your total health and life!

Patricia Bragg and *Paul C. Bragg*

Chapter 18

Treatments for Common Foot Conditions & Ailments

Find the Best Solution

We have compiled a list of some of the most common foot problems and solutions. However, there are many remedies for foot ailments, based on different medical theories. It may take additional research and some experimentation on your part to find the right solution for your particular foot problem. It is possible that the nature of your ailment will require you to treat it in ways other than the ones we have outlined here. As always, don't hesitate to seek a qualified foot doctor's opinion or to get a second or third opinion!

Achilles Tendinitis

Description: Achilles Tendonitis is a condition triggered by suddenly increasing running speed, by rapid running after a period of non-sporting activity and by not warming up and stretching before running. Another common cause of Achilles Tendonitis is over-pronation (like flat feet) when the foot arch collapses upon bearing too much weight, resulting in added stress being placed on the Achilles Tendon. **The Achilles Tendon is the largest tendon in the body, and the most frequently ruptured tendon by athletes and sports people.**

Symptoms: include pain in the morning during the first steps of the day. Pain after exercise, usually begins mildly and often becomes progressively worse, with sluggishness in the foot and leg movement.

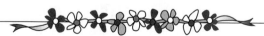

All of these foot conditions or ailments are caused or made worse by irritation or unnatural restriction of the feet. By following the Bragg Foot Care Program, which involves healthy diet, hygiene, exercise, and proper shoes, these common foot miseries can be curtailed or even prevented!

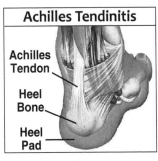

Achilles Tendinitis

Achilles Tendon

Heel Bone

Heel Pad

Best Treatment: rest, ample water, supplements and MSM. Stop sports and all activity for at least 2-4 weeks, and try swimming as a non-aggravating alternative to your regular exercise habits. If you are not improving, wear a foot boot to help restrict foot activity so it can heal.

Shoe Orthotics and Inner Shoe Cushions: These can help support damaged areas and provide some relief from discomfort. After a rest period, stretching should be introduced slowly to maintain flexibility and promote strength. *Surgery should be a last resort and only after wise cautious advice.*

Preventative Steps: Always walk, stretch and warm up before running. Make increases in running speed gradual – in increments of no more than 10% per week. Always choose running footwear carefully and replace regularly. For more ideas and info see web: *www.foot.com/info/cond_achillies_tendonitis.jsp*

(166) Achilles Tendinitis: Inflammation and Pain

If you have pain behind the heel, the area where the Achilles Tendon inserts into the heel bone may be inflamed.

To reduce inflammation after injury or activity, try the combination of rest, an ice pack (when there is swelling) and pain relief cream. Doing this will minimize tissue damage and reduce inflammation.

Blood carries the nutrients, oxygen and antibodies to the injured tissues to help repair and rebuild. Research shows that *electromagnetic energy* is an effective treatment for stimulating the blood flow to the tendons, ligaments and muscles. ***Electromagnetic energy*** is a waveform that is absorbed by the tendons, muscles and ligaments. Absorption of this energy translates to heat and that increases the blood flow to that area to speed up the body's healing process, clear the area of toxins and help reduce inflammation. This process is known as STR (Soft Tissue Repair Therapy). Please recognize that healing is a process.

Arthritis: Effects Millions

Arthritis is the umbrella term for a complex of diseases which cause the swelling and inflammation of the cartilage and lining of the joints, as well as an increase in joint fluid. The feet are particularly susceptible to arthritis because of the weight they bear and because each foot has so many potentially vulnerable joints.

Almost 60 million Americans are afflicted by this painful disease. Arthritis is primarily prevalent in those over 50, but now has victims of all ages, even children. There is some evidence to suggest that it might be hereditary in some manifestations, however, symptoms may appear through viral and bacterial infections – for example the organisms present in gonorrhea, pneumonia and Lyme disease can cause inflammations in the joints. Injuries, especially ignored injuries may lead to arthritic symptoms, and more often in the feet, where injuries most often can go untreated. Although seemingly unrelated, bowel disorders such as colitis and ileitis may also be accompanied by arthritic symptoms in the ankles and toe joints.

It is important to see a Podiatrist if you notice any of these symptoms in the feet: swelling, recurring pain, tenderness, redness or heat in a joint; early morning stiffness, limited joint motion and appearance of rashes and growths on the skin.

Osteoarthritis: Can Affect the Foot

Description: There are more than one hundred varieties of arthritis of which Osteoarthritis, or degenerative joint disease, is the most common form. Osteoarthritis usually develops gradually with age, as wear and tear on bones sees the cartilage covering become worn and frayed.

Symptoms: can include swelling or stiffness in the joint, tenderness or pain, reduced ability to move, walk or bear weight, and inflammation. Occasionally joint injuries can even cause the sudden onset of pain.

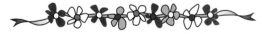

 Success is the sum of small efforts –
repeated day in and day out. – Robert Collier

Causes: Osteoarthritis can develop months or years after an injury. Obesity can exacerbate symptoms as excess weight accelerates deterioration of cartilage.

Treatments: include pads or arch supports (orthotics), canes or braces to support the joints, physical therapy, custom shoes, and weight control. Also wear shoes that fit properly and feel really comfortable. Exercise can help keep your feet pain-free, strong and flexible. Try the *Healthy Feet* and *Toe Exercises* on page 152.

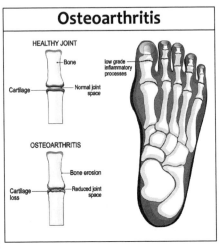

Rheumatoid Arthritis: of the Foot & Toes

Description: Rheumatoid Arthritis (RA) is the most crippling and serious form of arthritis. It is a complex, systematic disorder which affects multiple joints over the entire body. RA causes an over-activity of synovium – the lining that lubricates the joints and makes it easier to move. It swells and becomes inflamed, destroying the joint, as well as ligaments and other tissues that support it. The toes can twist and stiffen into positions called hammertoe or claw toe. As RA affects the various systems in the body, one may simultaneously experience fatigue, fever, loss of appetite and weight loss. Women are 3-4 times more likely to suffer from RA than men.

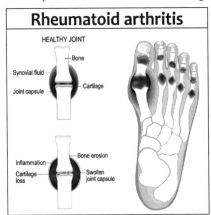

Rheumatoid arthritis is not an isolated disease of the bones and joints. It affects tissues throughout the body, causing damage to the blood vessels, nerves, and tendons. Deformities of the hands and feet are the more obvious signs of RA. In about 20% of patients, foot and ankle symptoms are the first signs of the disease. – orthoinfo.aaos.org

Symptoms: 90% of RA sufferers experience symptoms in their feet, ankles, knees, hips, hands, wrists and elbows. Most common symptoms are pain, stiffness and swelling. RA usually appears in the same joint in both feet.

Causes: The exact cause of RA is not know. Some people may be more prone to develop the disease because of family heredity. Some doctors say that it takes a chemical or environmental "trigger" to activate the disease in people who are genetically inclined.

Natural Treatments: Although it is said there is no cure for Rheumatoid Arthritis, there are treatment options to help manage pain and to stay active for a fulfilling life. Treatments may relieve symptoms, but might not stop progression of the disease.

- **REST** – Limit activities that make the pain worse. Biking or swimming are exercises that allow you to maintain health yet limit the impact load on the foot.
- **ICE** – the most painful area of the foot for 20 minutes. Can be done 3-4 times a day. Best done after exercising.
- **ORTHOTICS:** A shoe insert is a very effective tool to minimize pressure on prominent bones in the foot.

Athlete's Foot

Description: Athlete's Foot is a skin disease or condition, usually occurring between the toes, caused by a fungus which thrives in warm, moist conditions. The fungus proliferates on the feet because shoes create the ideal dark and humid environment. Swimming pools, showers and locker rooms are also breeding grounds for the fungi, and it is in such places that it is transferred from one person to another. Athlete's foot is so named because the fungal infection is most common among athletes. Millions suffer from it who frequent gyms, swimming pools, and the like.

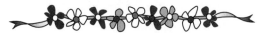

Rheumatoid Arthritis affects approximately 1.5 million people in the US. Women are affected more often than men, with a ratio of up to 3 to 1. Symptoms most commonly develop between the ages of 40 and 60.
– see web: ortholnfo.aaos.org

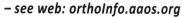

Symptoms: include itching, stinging or burning, scaly, inflamed, cracked skin and blisters. Also skin redness, rash, inflammation and discoloration and crumbling nails. When the blisters break and the raw underskin is exposed then the pain and discomfort increases! If the infection is scratched, it can spread to other parts of the foot, the soles and toenails, as well as to other body parts such as the underarms and groin. Athlete's foot can also be spread to other areas of the body by contaminated towels, clothing and bed sheets too.

Causes: Our body is normally the host to a variety of micro-organisms, including bacteria, mold-like fungi and yeast-like fungi. Some of these micro-organisms are useful to our body, but others may cause infections. Fungal skin infections are caused by microscopic fungi that can live on the skin. Athlete's Foot is the most common and most persistent of fungal (tinea) infections. Athlete's Foot may occur in association with other fungal skin infections such as ringworm or jock itch. Mold-like fungi live on dead tissues of hair, nails and outer skin layers and thrive in warm, moist areas of the body. Poor hygiene, prolonged moist skin and minor skin or nail injuries are also factors that can induce Athlete's Foot. Athlete's Foot is contagious! It can be spread through items such as shoes, socks, shower stalls and pool side surfaces of spas, clubs, gyms, summer camps, etc.

Expert Advice on Banishing Athlete's Foot

To avoid contracting the fungus, avoid walking barefoot in communal showers (wear rubber sandals). To control symptoms, wear light shoes or flip flops, change socks frequently and use cornstarch to reduce any perspiration.

Athlete's foot commonly occurs in people whose feet have become very sweaty while confined within tight-fitting shoes.

Develop a strong immune system. A weakened immune system puts you at risk for developing Athlete's Foot. Get enough sleep every night. Eat a balanced diet of organic fruits and veggies. Spend time outdoors, in the sunshine to get your vitamin D3. Manage stress and anxiety through exercise, prayer and meditation. – WikiHow.com/Get-Rid-of-Foot-Fungus

If you have Athlete's Foot, using self-care can help you banish the problem. Follow the foot soaking suggestions below and otherwise always keep feet clean and dry; always wear clean cotton or wool socks, change daily; wear shoes made of natural material such as leather or canvas and best to alternate shoes daily. Shoes then have time to dry completely between wearings; reduce perspiration by using cornstarch powder. When you are infected with Athlete's Foot, it's good to change bed sheets and clothing often to prevent the infection from spreading.

Treatment Tips to Help Banish Athlete's Foot:

- Soak feet daily in raw, organic apple cider vinegar ($1/2$ cup) and warm water in shallow pan to help banish athlete's foot and fungus. Repeat daily until subsides (*ideal while reading or watching TV*).

- Soak your feet in warm water with 2 Tbsps each of salt and raw, organic apple cider vinegar in a shallow pan.

- Apply a baking soda paste to fungus between the toes for 1-2 hours. Prepare the paste with a few drops of raw, organic apple cider vinegar to 1 Tbsp. of baking soda. Wear white cotton socks after applying. After treatment: rinse, dry and dust area with cornstarch (*optional add $1/3$ tsp garlic powder*).

- Let your feet air out during an acute bout as much as possible without walking barefoot (wear sandals).

- Avoid walking barefoot. Carry a pair of pool sandals with you to the gym, locker room, hotel pool or any other public place. Avoid walking barefoot even in your own home. These measures will help to prevent re-infection.

- Avoid sweat. Fungus loves moisture and heat. Keep your feet as dry as possible. Pour a dash of cornstarch powder on your feet before putting on your socks. Make sure to change your socks frequently.

Athlete's foot can lead to complications in some cases.
Mild complications include an allergic reaction to the fungus,
which can lead to blistering on the feet or hands. It's also possible
for the fungal infection to return after treatment.

Blisters: On Your Feet

Description: Blisters are irritated areas which are very tender and filled with either air or fluid just under the skin.

Symptoms: Severe redness, swelling, soreness, pus, or even pain at the site.

Causes: Blisters are caused by an ill-fitting shoe rubbing against the affected area of the foot. They frequently occur when new shoes are worn and can be prevented by going barefoot when possible, wearing thick enough stockings or socks, or by flexing stiff areas of the shoe prior to wearing them. Remember, if a shoe requires that much breaking in, it didn't fit right in the first place! Buy shoes cautiously!

Treatment & Prevention: In general, do not pop blisters. This can increase irritation and sometimes promote infection. It's better to wait things out and keep the tender area protected when wearing shoes.

If it's a small blister, you can disinfect the area and pop it and let the fluid drain out. Here are some details to help you properly care for your blister: Use soap and water to thoroughly clean your hands and the blister. Then, clean off the blister with a little bit of rubbing alcohol or some iodine. Gently rub the blister to see if it will pop. If it does not, consider soaking the blister in warm water with apple cider vinegar for 30 minutes and gently rub again. Rub a little antibiotic ointment on the area after popping, then put a bandage over it.

You want to make sure there is no infection going on and that it's not actually an ulceration. For a person with diabetes, you should have it drained by a doctor.

Also exposure to air will speed heal blisters and let Mother Nature take its course. Blisters can be avoided if you are sensitive enough to feel the affected area beginning to become irritated. Remove or change shoes, or at least cover affected area with a band-aid or a cushioning "second skin" product such as moleskin.

Paying your feet the attention they deserve by choosing the right shoes and socks can help keep your feet healthy and blister-free.

Bunions: A Common Foot Disorder

Bunions

Bunion of the big toe

Bunion of the small toe

Description: A bunion is a large visible bump on the joint which connects the big toe to the foot (metatarsophalangeal or MTP joint). The toe is forced to bend towards the other toes causing an enlargement of the bone. This is a painful condition, as the joint carries much of the bodies weight. The pain can become chronic if left untreated! The second toe may be pushed out of alignment and arthritis may also develop. A smaller painful lump on the outside of the foot at the base of the little toe is called a **bunionette**. It should be treated in the same way as a big toe bunion.

Symptoms: Bunions begin with a leaning of the big toe, gradually changing the angle of the bones over the years and slowly producing the characteristic bump, which becomes increasingly prominent. Symptoms usually appear at the later stages, although some people never have symptoms. Symptoms occur most often when wearing shoes that crowd the toes, such as high heels. This may explain why women are more likely to have symptoms than men. In addition, spending a long time on your feet can aggravate the symptoms of bunions. More common symptoms, which occur at the site of the bunion, may include: pain or soreness; inflammation and redness; a burning sensation; and possible numbness.

Causes: are often from wearing tight, constricting shoes, boots and high heels, and more common in women than men. Certain foot types are more prone to developing a bunion. Sadly over 50% of women over 65 in the U.S. have bunions and foot problems.

Bunions are very common. While over-the-counter bunion pads and pain relievers ease symptoms, you should see a healthcare provider. Treatments can reduce pain and stop bunion symptoms from getting worse. – clevelandclinic.org

173

Even though foot problems and faulty foot mechanics can be hereditary, it is bad habits such as the wearing of narrow, ill-fitting pointed shoes that is the cause of most bunions in 90% of cases. Other causes are congenital deformities, neuromuscular disorders and foot injuries. Most ballet dancers are prone to developing bunions and arthritis sufferers, people with flat feet or low heel arches and even cowboy boot wearers are also at serious risk!

Treatments: Choose comfortable shoes that conform to the size of your foot, preferably with a wide instep and broad toe box (see pages 204-205). **Never force your foot into a shoe that is too small, too short and too tight!!!** Avoid all sharply pointed shoes and heels of more than 2 inches.

If you already have a bunion, you can apply a non-medicated bunion pad around the bony protuberance. Shoe inserts may be helpful for reducing pain and for preventing symptoms from worsening. If the bunion becomes inflamed, apply ice packs several times daily to reduce the swelling and pain. Avoid activity that causes bunion pain, including standing for long periods of time. It's wise to seek a professional podiatrist's advice if the pain continues.

Be Cautious with All Bunion Surgery

Should **bunion** surgery be required, several procedures are offered. In a simple bunionectomy the surgeon removes just the bony protuberance. More severe cases might require a serious and complex procedure involving the cutting of the bone and joint realignment. Bunion surgery is generally done on the same day, on an outpatient basis. However, recovery can be a slow process! **Get at least three opinions from board certified orthopedic doctors!** For more surgery and foot info: *orthoInfo.aaos.org* or *www.apma.org*

The treatment of diseases should go to the root cause, and most often it is found in severe dehydration from lack of sufficient pure, distilled water, plus an unhealthy diet and lifestyle!

He who wears the shoe, best knows where it pinches.
– Norwegian saying

What is Tightrope Bunionectomy?

Traditional bunion surgery may require six to eight weeks of recovery time, but a newer outpatient surgery can have you back on your feet right away with no need to wait for the bone to heal, and minimal scarring.

Tightrope bunionectomy is a relatively new procedure using a special suture material called "fiber wire" to bind the first and second metatarsals of the foot together into proper alignment. Holes are drilled through the first and second metatarsals and two sets of fiber wire are passed through the openings and anchored on either side. The surgeon uses x-ray guidance to ensure the desired alignment, allowing a level of correction not possible with other surgeries. Tightrope bunionectomy is much less painful than traditional surgery.

Advantages of the TightRope Bunionectomy include:
- Allows for immediate weight bearing
- Prevents recurrence of deformity
- Faster healing time
- More rapid return to normal activity
- Less post-operative pain
- Bone removal from the foot is not required

Complications of the TightRope Bunionectomy are:
- The bunion can come back
- Bone fractures and wound infections
- Excessive bleeding or developing a blood clot
- Anesthetic complications
- Toe numbness

Following the TightRope Bunionectomy Surgery you will be able to walk immediately (with special post-operative shoes). The stitches are removed after two or three weeks and most patients should recover after three to four weeks.

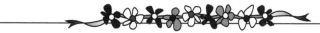

Prevention is always better than the treatment!

 If you want to change the world, start with yourself.
– Mahatma Gandhi

Our habits, good or bad, are something we can control. – Dr. E.J. Stieglitz

Calluses: on the Foot

Description: Calluses are patches of rough, dry, dead and hardened skin that may form on the ball of foot, heel and outside of the big toe or on other flat areas. Some have centers known as nucleations which can be painful when pressed.

Causes: calluses are formed due to continual friction or pressure from tight fitting or high heeled and pointed shoes. Also being obese, having flat feet or a lack of sufficient fat padding on the feet are possible causes.

Calluses can also be caused by bad walking habits and bad posture when standing. This moves the feet out of line with the shoe, or promotes slipping or tilting of the shoe with respect to the foot. Again, the difficulty may be either with the shoes, a misaligned foot, or your posture. **Calluses are natures way of protecting an area beneath skin.** Calluses also appear on the hands for example, but in a useful protective capacity. Many musicians who play stringed instruments find it a painful occupation until thick calluses appear on the fingertips to protect them. In countries where people go barefoot much of the time, a thick and useful layer of callus forms on the feet to offer protection! However in western societies where the wearing of shoes is normal, calluses are usually symptoms of mechanical problems, and can continue to aggravate and cause discomfort until the problem is corrected!

How to Treat Foot Calluses

If your shoes are causing calluses, either cushion the insides or buy new shoes. Calluses may be painful and get worse through continued irritation. If the problem, then is in the feet themselves, changing shoes will not be the total answer. What's necessary is following the *Bragg Foot Care Program* faithfully 100%, and also improving your posture and walking strides.

Immediate relief from a callus may be obtained by placing a thin piece of moleskin directly over the callus, but separated from it by cotton or gauze. When you remove the moleskin each day, slowly pull the moleskin off. Never rip it off, or you may end up with a bleeding callus!

Opinion is divided among the experts whether to use a pumice stone or callus wand to file down a callus, *both are okay*. Here's how: soak your feet in a shallow pan of warm water with 3 Tbsps. raw, organic apple cider vinegar, then dry well and gently rub away the dead skin with a pumice stone or callus wand. Please be gentle and don't overdo and irritate the area!!! *Caution: Feet do need some natural fat padding!*

Many people try to alleviate the pain caused by calluses by cutting or trimming them with a razor blade or knife. This is very dangerous and can worsen the condition resulting in unnecessary injuries. Diabetics especially should never try this type of treatment. To relieve the excessive pressure that leads to callus formation, weight should be redistributed equally with the use of an orthotic. An effective orthotic transfers pressure away from the "hot spots" or high pressured areas to allow the callus to heal. The orthotic should be made with materials that absorb shock and shear (friction) forces. Women are wise to stop wearing high heeled shoes. **Remember foot surgery should be the very last resort.**

Corns: Caused by Repeated Rubbing

Description: Corns are the build up of small circles of hard, thickened skin cells, usually located on the top or inside of the toe or between the toes. Since corns are cone-shaped, with the tip penetrating into the tender tissue underneath, they can become especially painful.

Soft corns: are usually found between toes, often in pairs, facing one another and stay soft due to perspiration. They are caused when the bones of the opposing toes rub against one another. *Seed corns:* are small and often develop in groups. They are frequently found on the soles and may be a result of irritation from protruding shoe tacks. Sometimes a corn will develop within a callus, creating double trouble!

People with damaged sweat glands, scars or warts on their feet are more likely to get corns. Also, people with diabetes or other conditions that cause poor circulation to the feet have a higher risk of complications from corns. In such cases, getting your corn treated by a foot doctor is highly recommended. – Top10HomeRemedies.com

Causes: A very common ailment, corns are formed by friction against a tight fitting shoe for example. The irritation increases the blood supply to the area and the cells grow in an accelerated fashion, causing a corn. If they are left unchecked corns can become inflamed and extremely sore.

How to Treat Foot Corns

The development of corns does not necessarily mean the fault is with the shoe. Your posture or gait may be pushing a perfectly good shoe out of shape and your aching foot with it. Do all your shoes produce irritation in the same places? If so, this is a fairly sure indication that you need to become more aware of your feet and their misalignment.

Beware of over-the-counter medications which claim to remove the *root* of the problem, because corns have no root! Incidentally, many corn cure products contain an acid which eats away the corn and also the surrounding healthy tissue and can cause ulcerations. Always use with caution! If you want to use a corn pad to obtain immediate relief, make certain it doesn't contain an oval area with acid in it. If it does, cut out this oval area. You can make a horseshoe-shaped pad and stick it just behind and around the corn. The pad should not rub up against the corn, for that will just increase the irritation.

A better idea is to use a simple spot band-aid. Place band-aid with sterile gauze spot directly over the corn. If you have a soft corn, you can also wrap soft material such as lamb's wool around the toe to help cushion. Don't wrap it too tight, as this restricts the circulation.

You can also soak your feet in a shallow pan with 3 Tbsps. organic apple cider vinegar and water regularly to soften the corns and use a pumice stone to lightly brush away dead skin cells as needed. You can wear a corn pad over the problem area to relieve the pressure. Applying organic extra-virgin olive oil will help keep skin soft, but corn removing ointments that contain toxic acid can damage healthy skin. They should never be used by pregnant women or by people who are diabetic or who have poor circulation.

For both corns and calluses, remove any dressing and wash the area each evening. It's best to leave the area uncovered at night and allow Mother Nature to do her healing. *Do not under any circumstance use a razor blade to try to cut out the corn or callus.* This will make things far worse. If the problem is that severe, consult your foot doctor! He or she will be able to help control corns by carefully trimming them, however this should not be done at home, especially by diabetics! Remember, corns and calluses will disappear if you stop wearing ill-fitting tight shoes.

Prevention: of foot corns is relatively simple. Always wear well fitted shoes with deep and wide toe boxes. Buy shoes made from materials which breathe and are flexible such as leather, canvas, etc., wear cotton or wool socks and wash your feet often, drying well afterwards. Go barefoot as often as possible and your feet will thank you, but diabetics wear socks!

Diabetes and Foot Problems

Description: Diabetes is a disease which brings about the inability of the body to produce insulin, or convert sugars, starches and other foods into energy. High blood sugar levels are a result and the long term effects. Many complications can be associated with diabetes. Diabetes can disrupt the vascular system, affecting many areas of the body such as the eyes, heart, kidneys, nerves, blood vessels, legs, and feet. People with diabetes should pay special attention to their feet.

Symptoms: include slow to heal wounds, blurred vision, dry skin, fatigue, excessive weight loss, hunger and thirst, frequent urination and even numbness of the hands and feet.

Corns and calluses were described by Hippocrates, Father of Medicine, who recognized the need to physically reduce hard skin, followed by removal of cause. He invented skin scrapers for this purpose and these were the original scalpels. A Roman Scientist and Philosopher, Aulus Cornelius Celsus was probably responsible for giving corns their name.

The warning signs of type 2 diabetes can be so mild that you don't notice them. Some people don't find out they have it until they get problems from long-term damage caused by the disease. – www.webmd.com

Causes: unknown, but we strongly feel it is lifestyle, diet, habits and processed, high-sugar foods and beverages, that most often trigger the problems! Most doctors say there is no known cure, but Dr. Dean Ornish, (*ornish.com*) says with dietary changes and exercise, diabetics can improve and may keep serious symptoms at bay! Self-testing for blood sugar levels is an important measure in warding off complications!

Diabetes affects over 30 million Americans and is classified into two different types. **Type 1** which does occurs most frequently in children and adolescents and is caused by the inability of the pancreas to produce necessary insulin. **Type 2** or adult onset diabetes, affects 90-95% of cases, who have to inject insulin or take oral medication to control the disease.

Of the millions of Americans with diabetes, 25% will develop foot problems related to the disease. Diabetic foot problems include: sores or ulcers, neuropathy, poor circulation, and deformities such as bunions or hammer toes.

Diabetes and Foot Ulcers

Foot ulcers are a common complication of diabetes. Ulcers are formed as a result of skin tissue breaking down and exposing the layers underneath. They're most common under your big toes and the balls of your feet, and they can affect your feet down to the bones. Foot ulcers and gangrene effect about 15% of diabetics and sadly between 15% and 25% require amputation with a 50% likelihood of further amputations, within five years. *(Dr. Linus Pauling saved limbs with a daily 2-3 hour slow I.V. drip of 30-50g of Vitamin "C.")*

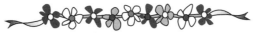

Beware, physicians are not usually reimbursed for efforts to prevent foot problems, therefor it is important to care for your own feet. Make sure there are no ulcers, which are extremely hard to heal when you have diabetes. Watch out for feelings of pins and needles and numbness – diabetic nerve damage caused by restricted blood flow in the small vessels of the feet. Poor circulation, lack of sensation, wounds and ulcers of the feet, can worsen without the person's knowledge and are difficult to treat due to the lack of blood circulation.

Ulceration may also be caused by poorly fitting shoes or something as simple as a rubbing stocking seam. As skin sensation is diminished, a wound can quickly develop unnoticed. A foot physician (podiatrist) can help prevent and treat such wounds. There are remarkable scientific developments – new substances, which have the feel and texture of human skin which may be applied to the problem area. There are also many preventative measures the diabetic can take to diminish the risk of ulcers and other complications. Careful inspection of the diabetic foot on a regular basis is one of the easiest, least expensive and most effective measures for preventing foot complications.

Treating Diabetic Foot Ulcers

The primary goal in treating foot ulcers is to obtain healing as soon as possible. The faster the healing, the less chance of an infection. There are several key factors in the appropriate treatment of a diabetic foot ulcer:

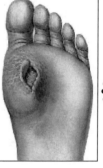

Foot Ulcer

- Prevent an infection
- Take pressure off of the area, called "off-loading"
- Remove dead skin and tissue, called "debridement"
- Apply medication or dressings to the ulcer
- Manage blood glucose and other health problems

Not all ulcers will get infected; however, if your podiatrist diagnoses an infection, a treatment program of antibiotics, wound care, and possibly hospitalization will be urgent!

A foot ulcer is typically a painful inconvenience to most people, but to a person with diabetes it could mean an infection, or worse, an amputation.

A drug delivered through a skin patch that not only helps foot wounds heal better, but also prevents those wounds from recurring, has been developed by researchers. "The use of the LeucoPatch is associated with significant enhancement of healing of hard-to-heal foot ulcers in people with diabetes." – The Lancet (Diabetes and Endocrinology). See websites: www.sciencedaily.com and www.3cpatch.com

Diabetic Neuropathy is A Common Serious Complication of Diabetes

Diabetic neuropathy is a type of nerve damage that can occur if you have diabetes. High blood sugar can injure nerves throughout your body. Diabetic neuropathy most often damages nerves in your legs and feet. Of the millions of Americans with diabetes, 25% will develop foot problems related to the disease. Diabetic neuropathy can cause insensitivity or a loss of ability to feel pain, heat, and cold. Diabetics suffering from neuropathy can develop minor cuts, scrapes, blisters, or pressure sores that they may not be aware of due to this insensitivity. If these minor injuries are left untreated, complications may result and lead to ulceration and possibly even amputation. Neuropathy can also cause deformities such as bunions and hammer toes. It is very important for diabetics to take the necessary precautions to prevent all foot related injuries. Due to the consequences of neuropathy, daily observation of the feet is critical. **When a diabetic patient takes the necessary preventative foot-care measures, they reduce the risks of serious foot conditions and amputations.**

182

Diabetes and Poor Circulation Problems

Diabetes often leads to peripheral vascular disease that inhibits a person's blood circulation. With this condition, there is a narrowing of arteries that frequently leads to significantly decreased circulation in the lower part of the legs and feet. Poor circulation contributes to diabetic foot problems by reducing the amount of oxygen and nutrition supplied to skin and other tissues, causing injuries to heal poorly. Poor circulation can also lead to swelling and dryness of the foot. **Preventing foot complications is more critical for the diabetic patient because poor circulation impairs the healing process and can lead to ulcers, infection, and other serious foot conditions.**

The skin found in the palms of the hands and the soles of the feet is thickest because the epidermis contains an extra layer, the stratum lucidum. – www.ncbi.nlm.nih.gov

Basic Preventative Care for Diabetic Feet

1. Wash your feet morning and night with mild soap and lukewarm water (never hot – test the water with thermometer to make sure). Diabetics should not do foot soaks as skin can become soft, cracked and more vulnerable. With a soft towel dry your feet carefully, and use cornstarch or tea tree powder to keep feet dry.

2. Check feet and toes daily for sores, cuts, red spots and bruises (use a mirror if needed). Inspect the toenails for changes in coloration or thickening.

3. Keep your body as healthy and fit as possible and your weight normal to reduce any likelihood of future diabetic complications! Many diabetics tend to overeat and become dangerously overweight! *www.aofas.org*

4. If you are a smoker, stop now to reduce the risks of circulatory problems, and don't drink alcohol! Drinking accelerates the development of diabetic problems and causes numb feet, creating a possible serious risk of undetected injury.

5. Exercise is an excellent way to improve your circulation and keep weight down. Walking is the best exercise for diabetics, especially after meals. Wearing comfortable shoes is a must.

6. Wear thick, seamless, soft socks and choose well fitted shoes that protect your feet. High heels, boots and all shoes with pointed toes must be avoided! Don't wear tight, constricting leg wear. Don't walk barefoot, not even indoors – wear socks, and especially not outdoors, to avoid cuts and any possible infection! Always check insides of shoes before putting them on. Make sure there are no foreign objects in shoes.

7. Diabetics don't try to remove calluses or corns yourself as many preparations can burn, even scar the skin.

8. Trim toenails straight across, avoid cutting in the corners. Use an emery board to gently smooth any rough corners.

9. Have regular foot checkups with your foot doctor.

10. Take care of your diabetes. Make healthy lifestyle choices to keep blood sugar as close to normal as possible.

Flat Feet or Fallen Arches

Description: Over 20% of Americans have flat feet and they are seldom inherited. Flat feet is what happens when foot arches collapse due to several factors, including obesity, pregnancy and repeated contact of foot base with hard surfaces. Studies show children (in their first 6 years) who go barefoot more often have better arches and are less likely to develop flat feet. As foot framework caves in, extra stress is placed on other parts of the foot. Often some people with flat feet don't experience discomfort immediately, and some never suffer from any discomfort at all. However, when pain does develop, then walking becomes awkward and causes increased strain on the feet and calves!

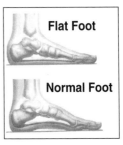

Symptoms: In people with fallen arches, the normal pressure of walking shifts to other parts of the feet. If not treated properly, this can cause prolonged discomfort, pain and in some cases heel spurs, plantar fasciitis and tendonitis, among other ailments, may result.

Causes: Flat feet can be attributed to:
- Wearing shoes with poor arch support
- Excessive walking or standing on high heels
- Muscle damage caused by excessive strain on the feet
- Ruptured or over-stretched tendons
- Abnormality at birth
- The risk of developing flat feet also increases with diabetes, pregnancy, obesity and ageing.

Treatments: are dependent on the severity of the condition and the underlying cause. We suggest the following:

- Orthotic arch supports (such as Dr. Scholls).
  They should be supportive and feel comfortable in the arch area. Always choose footwear with care to ensure comfortable and a proper fit.
- *Bragg Foot Exercises* (pages 152-154)
- Ice and compression to reduce pain and swelling
- Physical Therapy

Flat feet can cause a variety of painful symptoms. Many have been relieved by orthotic supports for decades.

Foot Odors Can Be Embarrassing

Description, Symptoms and Causes: There are two principal reasons for malodorous smelly feet. First, feet sweat and second they are usually encased in shoes for most of the day.

Bacteria thrives in socks and shoes where a combination of darkness and heat which can reach 102°F, creating the perfect breeding ground! The greater the amount of moisture, the more bacteria is generated. In turn bacteria produces a substance called *isovaleric acid* which is the source of most foot odors. People with *Hyperhidrosis* (abnormal excessive sweating) should see their doctor if their heavy sweating is accompanied by lightheadedness, chest pain or nausea. Wear well-ventilated shoes, sandals or sneakers with breathing holes to allow feet to breathe and be healthy! Also go barefoot at home or whenever possible.

Foot Hygiene Important to Eliminate Odors

It is important to practice good foot hygiene to keep bacteria levels down. Soak your feet daily in warm soapy vinegar water for about 10 minutes. Dry thoroughly afterwards. Apply cornstarch powder. Change shoes and socks everyday. Alternate shoes, don't wear the same pair two days in a row. Wear shoes that are made from materials that allow your feet to breathe such as leather or canvas. It's best to avoid nylon socks and plastic shoes.

You may also try soaking your feet in strong black tea for 30 minutes per day for a week. The tannic acid in black tea will help kill the bacteria. Use four tea bags per pint of water, boil the mixture for 15 minutes, then add two quarts of cool water. Soak your feet in the warm brew. See page 150 for tips on how to do away with smelly feet! For more foot care info, check out web: *orthoInfo.aaos.org*

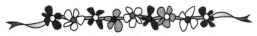

You can neutralize the isovaleric acid with an alkaloid like baking soda. Sprinkle half to a whole tablespoon of plain baking soda into each shoe and leave them overnight.

Gout: Common in the Big Toe

Description: Gout is a form of arthritis. Millions (mostly men), suffer from this painful condition. Gout is a disorder that results from the buildup of uric acid in the tissues or joints and usually affects the joint of the big toe, but also can affect joints throughout the body.

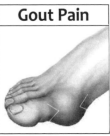

Gout Pain

Symptoms: An attack of gout can be miserable. Some symptoms to look for are: intense pain that comes on suddenly – often in the middle of the night or in the early morning. Also look for signs of inflammation such as redness, swelling and warmth over the joint.

Causes: Uric acid is present in the blood and eliminated in the urine, but for people who have gout, uric acid accumulates and crystallizes in the joints. Uric acid is the result of the breakdown of purines – chemicals found naturally in our bodies and food. Some people develop gout because their kidneys have difficulty eliminating normal amounts of uric acid, while others produce too much uric acid.

Risk Factors for Developing Gout

The tendency to accumulate uric acid is often inherited. Other factors that put a person at risk for gout include: high blood pressure, diabetes, obesity, alcohol, coffee, surgery, chemotherapy, stress and certain medications. Gout is most common in men aged 40-60 but can also occur in younger men and women.

How to Reduce Gout Attacks

Consuming foods and beverages that contain high levels of purines can trigger an attack of gout. Some foods contain more purines than others and have often been associated with an increase of uric acid. *Limit or avoid the following:* anchovies, mackerel, sardines, nuts roasted in oil, shellfish, red meat, organ meat (brains, kidney, liver, etc.), heavy sauces, coffee, alcohol, red wine, and beer. Stop all white sugar and refined flour products! Make sure to drink plenty of water and live The Bragg Healthy Lifestyle!

Natural Foot Treatments for Gout Pain

Conservative foot treatments to reduce gout include: a healthy diet, fasting, weight control and wearing proper shoes. Try keeping the inflamed area mobile and more flexible. Exercising, especially in a pool is particularly beneficial. In water you weigh less, put less strain on the joints and are more flexible. It's also very important to maintain good body posture and foot balance to reduce stress on the joints.

Herbal teas such as Yarrow, Willow Bark, Dandelion and Burdock are known to help relieve gout pains. Taking Vitamin C, CoQ10 and MSM is helpful. Garlic (fresh is best) boosts the immune system and helps reduce pain. A paste made of cayenne oil and wintergreen oil applied to sore areas helps relieve pain and inflammation.

The symptoms of gout usually resolve in three to ten days with treatment. If gout symptoms continue, or if repeated attacks occur, see your physician for maintenance treatments. Over time a build-up of uric acid can cause damage to the joint.

187

Apple Cider Vinegar is a Great Way to Get Rid of Gout!

Apple cider vinegar is a great natural cure for this ailment. Make sure it's organic, raw and unfiltered and contains the "mother enzyme" which have the maximum health benefits and are referred to as strand-like structures. This acetic acid proves to be immensely beneficial in reducing pain in the joints due to gout and the malic acid content. ACV helps neutralize uric acid collected in joints, dissolving the uric acid crystals and flushing them out of your body. Apple cider vinegar is high in amino acids which has an antibiotic effect by reducing toxicity and excess water. It eases the gout pain by reducing inflammation and altering the pH levels in your body. It's recommended to take apple cider vinegar at least 3 times a day (see ACV drink recipe page 40).

For effective gout topical treatment you can soak your affected foot for 30 minutes in a bucket of four cups of warm to hot water and one cup of vinegar.

Hammertoes

Description: Hammertoes are the bending of one or more of the 2nd to 5th toes at the middle joint. *Flexible Hammertoes* is the condition in early stages, because they are still moveable at the joint and more easily treatable with hammertoe splints, proper shoes and orthotics. If allowed

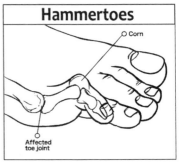

Hammertoes

O Corn

Affected toe joint

to develop into *Rigid Hammertoes* the situation becomes more serious. Joints become misaligned and immobile, the tendons tight, and often the only remaining recourse is toe surgery.

Symptoms: Common symptoms can include:
- Pain or irritation of affected toe when wearing shoes.
- Corns/calluses on the toe or on the ball of the foot.
- Inflammation, redness, or burning sensations.
- Contracture of the toe.

Causes: The most common cause of hammertoes is a muscle/tendon imbalance, which causes pressure on the joints and tendons, finally resulting in a contraction. The toe takes on a V, or hammer shape. A hammertoe may result if a toe is too long and is forced into a cramped position when a tight shoe is worn. The condition may also be hereditary, brought on by earlier trauma or even arthritis.

Treatment: Hammertoes don't go away by themselves. The first, most effective conservative treatment should be to wear shoes with soft, deep and roomy toe boxes (see pages 203-207). Wearing high heels should absolutely be avoided! A non-medicated hammertoe pad (*DrScholls.com*) may be applied around the bony prominence to decrease pressure on the area. If the hammertoe becomes inflamed, ice packs may be applied several times daily. A podiatric physician may also be able to suggest certain exercises to stretch and strengthen muscles such as picking objects up (pencils, marbles) off the floor with your toes.

Should all conservative measures fail, hammertoes can be corrected by surgery (please, get three opinions) which is usually carried out, using local anesthetic, on an outpatient basis.

Heel Fissures or Cracked Heels

Definition: Heel fissures, also known as cracked heels can be a simple cosmetic problem and a nuisance, but can also lead to serious medical problems. Heel fissures occur when the skin on the bottom, outer edge of the heel becomes hard, dry and flaky, sometimes causing deep fissures that can be painful or bleed. Heel fissures can lead to deep ulcers that can get infected. That's why preventing and treating heel fissures whenever possible is so important.

Symptoms: brown or yellow discoloration of the skin (which indicates the presence of callus), thickening of the skin around the crack or cracks, visible cracking or splitting of the skin on the heels. Also bleeding from the cracks and pain when putting pressure on the heels.

Causes: Heel fissures can affect anyone, but risk factors include: living in a dry climate; obesity; consistently walking barefoot or wearing sandals or open-backed shoes; and inactive sweat glands. Like many foot conditions, heel fissures can become more dangerous if they go untreated and become deep or infected. This is especially dangerous for people with diabetes.

Treatment and Prevention: Moisturizing the feet regularly can prevent heel fissures. Avoid going barefoot or wearing open-backed shoes, sandals or shoes with thin soles. Moisturizing the feet at least twice a day and wearing socks over moisturizer while sleeping can also help. Don't use harsh soaps, or soak your feet in very hot water. Exfoliate regularly using a gentle foot scrub, loofah or pumice stone to prevent the building of excess dead skin cells. *For infected fissures:* Using a mild topical ointment like *bacitracin* applied twice a day with a dressing is helpful. Take a Q-tip and 'work' the medication into the fissure itself. Because *bacitracin* is an ointment it will also help soften the area.

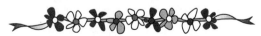

Lose weight to prevent cracked heels. Even small amounts of weight gain can add pressure to your heels. Pressure while walking, standing or running greatly increases when you gain weight. Not only will losing weight improve your foot health, it will be great for your entire well-being.

Heel Pain Syndrome

Description: Heel pain is a common condition in which weight bearing on the heel causes extreme discomfort. The pain can be sharp and originates deep within the foot. Heel pain usually occurs when the connective tissue – extending from the heel

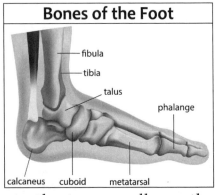

Bones of the Foot

fibula
tibia
talus
phalange
calcaneus   cuboid   metatarsal

bone, supporting the arch, to the toes – pulls on the bone at the heel and becomes irritated. When weight is applied to the foot the irritation can develop into an inflammation, causing severe pain.

Symptoms: Heel pain is usually worse in the morning or after sitting for long periods of time.

Cause: It's usually caused by walking gait abnormalities which place too much stress on the heel bone, or by heavy pounding of the feet on hard surfaces such as concrete, either while playing sports, or simply by wearing shoes which offer little or not sufficient cushioning. It can be caused by shoes with heels that are too low, a thinned out fat pad in the heel area, or from a sudden increase in activity.

Treatment: **Pain is nature's warning signal, telling us that if we don't pay attention to it, problems will follow!** Usually the heel pain will go away on its own accord if one refrains from the activities or shoes which caused the pain and when the foot is given rest!

To help alleviate heel pain, you can absorb the shock, provide cushioning and elevate the heel to transfer pressure. This can be done with a heel cup or an orthotic designed with materials that will help absorb shock. Also shoes with a firm heel counter, good arch support and appropriate heel height are the ideal choice.

Heel pain is most often caused by plantar fasciitis (see page 195), a condition that is sometimes also called heel spur syndrome when a spur is present (next page). Heel pain may also be due to other causes, such as a stress fracture, tendonitis, arthritis, nerve irritation or, rarely, a cyst.

Heel Spurs Are Not Spike-Shaped

Description: A heel spur develops as an abnormal growth of the heel bone. Calcium deposits form when the plantar fascia pulls away from the heel area, causing a bony protrusion, or heel spur to develop. It can extend up to half an inch on the inside of the heel. It is flat and wide in shape and is only visible using an x-ray.

Symptoms: Heel spurs can cause extreme pain in the rear of the foot, especially while standing or walking.

Causes: Heel spurs occur when the plantar fascia is strained over a long period of time. This stretching is usually the result of flat feet, but people with unusually high arches can also develop heel spurs. Sporting activity is another cause, as are shoes which offer inappropriate support, weight changes and obesity.

Treatment: The condition will generally improve greatly with rest. However, rest is a course of action which should be undertaken for short periods only, as muscular atrophy may result and may only contribute to the problem.

Other ways to treat heel spurs: Use an *ice pack* or cold compress on your foot for 10-15 minutes at a time. Or, roll a frozen water bottle under your foot. This method incorporates a bit of massage, relieving tightness in the bottom of your foot. You can also try *massaging* the arch of your foot to help relieve pain and promote mobility.

Inserts can be worn in your shoes for additional support and cushioning. Kinesiology tape can be used to improve arch and heel support.

Some find relief with using *night splints*. They are worn while sleeping to help keep the plantar fascia relaxed and prevent you from pointing your feet down.

Cryoultrasound Therapy may help treat pain due to both plantar fasciitis and heel spurs. This technique uses electromagnetic energy and cold therapy to relieve pain.

Other treatments include: losing weight, wearing shoes that have a cushioned heel that absorbs shock, and elevating the heel with the use of a heel cradle, heel cup, or orthotic. These provide extra comfort and cushion to the heel, and reduce the amount of shock. **As always, surgery should be a last resort.**

Ingrown Toenail

Description: Much confusion exists concerning ingrown toenails. The nail doesn't really *grow into* the flesh at either side. What happens is that the side flesh is forced into and over the sides of the nail.

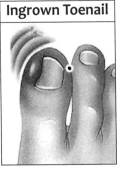

Ingrown Toenail

Symptoms: The area around the nail will become sore and tender, later possibly becoming infected and very painful. If left unattended the skin may begin to grow over the nail. If an ingrown nail causes a break in the skin, bacteria may enter and cause an infection, which is often marked by drainage and foul odor. However, even if the toe isn't painful, red, swollen, or warm – a nail that curves downward into the skin can progress into an infection. Usually the big toe is affected.

Causes: This extremely common ailment is often caused by trimming your toenails too short and rounding off the corner to match the shape of the toe while doing so. What happens is that this encourages the toenail to grow into the skin of the toe, often curling as it does so and embedding downwards. Other causes include: heredity; trauma to the nail, such as stubbing your toe or an object falling on your toe. Also improperly sized footwear (shoes that are tight or too short), or a nail condition such as a fungal infection or losing the nail.

192

Treatment: should be done as soon as it is recognized to prevent infection. Begin with soaking the foot in warm vinegar water for 5-10 minutes several times per day. This greatly relives irritation. Keep the foot dry during the rest of the day. Cleanliness is important. Don't attempt to cut down into nail groove on either side to relieve pressure. If you do, you may leave small

What you should know about home treatments: Don't cut a "V" notch in the nail. Contrary to what some people believe, this does not reduce the tendency for the nail to curve downward. Don't repeatedly trim nail borders. Repeated trimming does not change the way the nail grows, and can make the condition worse. Over-the-counter medications are ineffective. Topical medications may mask the pain, but they don't correct the underlying problem.

bony hooks or spicules on the nail that will cut into the flesh and cause painful, irritated flesh to form at the edge of the nail grooves. To relieve the soreness of the side grooves, gently work a little absorbent cotton or waxed dental floss between the nail and the flesh. If these measures do not give relief, or if other, more severe, nail problems develop, promptly see a podiatrist.

If excessive inflammation, swelling, pain and discharge are present the toenail is probably infected and should be treated by a physician. The nail may need to be partially removed. The doctor can surgically remove a portion of the nail, some of the soft tissues and even a part of the growth center. Surgery is effective in eliminating the nail edge from growing inward and cutting into the flesh.

How to Prevent Ingrown Toenails

If your shoes are too short or too tight, they may exert constant pressure on the toes, especially the big toe, causing ingrown toenails. To prevent this, make sure there is a half-inch of space between the longest toe and the front of the shoe, and that the toe box is not too narrow. Wear sandals if possible.

Proper cutting of the toenails is done straight across, without cutting down into the nail grooves. It used to be thought that ingrown toenails could be cured by cutting a wedge in the center of the nail, since the nail would then grow inward to fill the wedge. This is not true! The nail always grows straight out from the bottom, taking about 120 days to make the full trip out to cutting length.

Essential Oil to Prevent Infections of Ingrown Toenails

Don't apply essential oils directly to your skin without diluting with a carrier oil. Mix 2-3 drops of essential oil along with 1 teaspoon of a carrier oil (olive oil, jojoba). Then using a clean cotton ball coat the affected area of the toe. Make sure that you are only touching the area of your skin that is affected by the infection so that you don't spread the infection over healthy skin. This can help relieve pain and prevent infection. You may need to apply the oils 2-3 times per day over a period of several weeks to see results. Essential oils to try: Cinnamon; Thyme; Lemongrass; Peppermint; Eucalyptus; Tea tree; Lavender; and Oregano.

Morton's Neuroma

Definition: Morton's Neuroma is a common foot problem associated with pain, swelling and/or an inflammation of a nerve, usually at the ball of the foot between the 3rd and 4th toes.

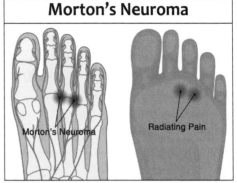

Morton's Neuroma

Morton's Neuroma

Radiating Pain

Symptoms: sharp pain just behind the 3rd and 4th toes (which can radiate to the other toes); burning; and lack of feeling in the affected area. Other symptoms are tingling or cramping in the fore-foot. It is commonly described as the awkward feeling of 'walking on a marble'.

Causes: It is caused by an abnormal function of the foot causing the bones to squeeze the nerve at this point.

The main factors that contribute to the formation of a neuroma are deformities such as flat feet or high arches, which place abnormal stress on the toe joints. The wearing of high heels, boots and constricting footwear that cause the toes to be squeezed together, promote injury and stress to the foot.

194

Treatment: The first step in treatment or prevention is to wear roomy and comfortable footwear that allow the bones to spread out and avoid high heels. Custom shoe orthotics may help to relieve pain by supporting and separating the bones. Foot soaks and massage are effective in temporary pain relief, as is rest. An ice pack (20 minutes on and off) may be applied to dull pain.

For more severe and long term cases, surgery may be necessary. The procedure to remove the enlarged nerve is usually carried out on an outpatient basis. The recovery time may be several weeks.

Other Conditions That Cause Similar Symptoms

There are other conditions that can mimic Morton's Neuroma pain. **Bursitis** in between the two metatarsal bones may put pressure on the nerve and cause pain. **Capsulitis** may also give similar symptoms. Also, a **Metatarsal Stress Facture** may create similar symptoms.

Plantar Fasciitis

Description: Plantar fasciitis, a very common diagnosis of heel pain. Plantar Fasciitis is an irritation or inflammation of the plantar fascia – the broad band of fibrous tissue that runs along the bottom surface of the foot, from the heel through midfoot and into the forefoot.

Symptoms: sharp pain directly under the heel – especially with the first few steps in the morning or after sitting for a while. Pain usually eases with walking or activity and comes back worsened after resting. Pain will gradually subside during the day and while sleeping.

Causes: Over-pronation (flat feet) can cause the plantar fascia to be excessively stretched and inflamed. Repetitive stresses or strain cause micro-tears in the plantar fascia, which become much larger with continual use. Other common causes can include: activity or training that is new or advanced too much or too quickly; standing for prolonged periods on concrete or hard surfaces; tight calf muscles; increased weight; and improper footwear.

Treatments: Rest your foot. Gentle stretches can help relieve and even prevent plantar fasciitis. Stretching your calves and the plantar fascia itself helps loosen your muscles and reduce heel pain. Do heel and foot muscle stretches. Wear shoes with good arch support and a cushioned orthotic pad such as Dr. Scholl's. You can also help your plantar fascia recover by stabilizing your foot with tape. This limits the amount that the ligament can move. It's important to take time off from certain exercises, like running, to give the plantar fascia time to heal. When you start running again, be sure to begin slowly. Stop and stretch while exercising to keep the pain from returning. Remember to stretch before beginning your workouts, too.

Stretching is the best treatment for plantar fasciitis. It may help to try to keep weight off your foot until the initial inflammation goes away. You can also apply ice to the sore area for 20 minutes three or four times a day to relieve your symptoms. Home exercises to stretch your Achilles tendon and plantar fascia are the mainstay of treatment and reduce the chance of recurrence.

Alternative Treatments for Plantar Fasciitis

Extracorporeal Shockwave Therapy (ESWT): Those with chronic plantar fasciitis may consider using this – shockwaves (see web: *eswtusa.com*) generated from a special ESWT device focused onto the targeted tissue. ESWT treatment is non-surgical and non-invasive. Shockwaves stimulate and reactivate healing by improving blood flow and nutrition to the injured area. ESWT also improves tissue healing – reducing pain and sensitivity to the heel area. Patients experience a short recovery period, with few or no side-effects. Most patients experience relief from pain right away. Results typically last forever.

Cold Laser Therapy: is a proven procedure that is non-invasive (no surgical incision). Cold Laser Therapy does not involve taking any medications. Cold laser is totally different from surgical laser. High power lasers are used to cut through tissue while low-power or "cold" lasers stimulate tissue repair and healing. No incision, no side effects! Cold laser may solve your heel or foot problems, and most importantly reduce your pain – even if you've been hurting for years. Cold Laser Therapy is totally painless and only takes a few minutes with each treatment session. Usually a series of treatments are needed, depending upon your injury.

Endoscopic Plantar Fasciotomy: can be used when physical therapy or custom orthotics fail to resolve your heel pain. With just a tiny incision, the endoscope is inserted into the heel area. The fiber-optic instrument transmits the image to a television monitor which allows a better view than the traditional surgical procedures. This endoscopic procedure is done under local anesthetic, and most patients are able to immediately put weight on the foot after surgery.

Two major causes of heel pain: Plantar Fasciitis and Achilles Tendinitis. The easiest way to figure out which one is causing your pain is by location. Generally speaking, if the pain is under your heel bone it is likely Plantar Fasciitis. If the pain is found at the back of the heel, in the achilles or toward the base of the achilles (the long cord that extends from your calf to your heel bone), then it is likely Achilles Tendinitis.

Toenail Fungus

Description: fungal infection of the nail may be present for years without causing discomfort, and for this reason often goes ignored. Toenail fungus is an infection underneath the surface of the nail caused by fungi. The result is thicker nails which are difficult to trim and make walking painful when wearing shoes. This may spread to other toenails, the skin and even the fingernails.

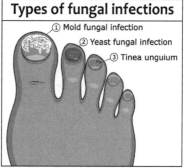

Types of fungal infections
① Mold fungal infection
② Yeast fungal infection
③ Tinea unguium

Symptoms: The toenails can often gradually change color and texture, becoming thick, dark and foul smelling. It may spread and cause the nails to thicken or crack.

Causes: The fungi thrive in damp environments such as showers, swimming pools and locker rooms – places where people are walking barefoot. It's best to wear bath sandals. Also injury to the nail bed may make it more susceptible to fungal infection. Those who have diabetes or circulatory problems are more prone to fungal nails.

Treatment: Soak and wash feet with apple cider vinegar and water (50/50 mix) on a daily basis (20 minutes), drying your feet thoroughly. Also try *Fungix™ Natural Nail Fungal Support*. It has 100% Pure Ingredients and is vegan friendly (web: *www.fungix.com*). Change socks and shoes more than once per day. You should visit a podiatrist when you notice any discoloration, thickening or deformity of your toenails. It is always best to catch any such infection in its early stages.

Prevention: Toenails should be cut straight across using nail clippers. Make sure instruments are disinfected. Cleanliness is the best prevention against infection. A mild infection may be temporarily suppressed by a daily vinegar cleansing routine (see above treatment). Wear well fitting shoes made of a material which breathes, such as leather and canvas. Avoid wearing tight socks to decrease moisture – wear socks made of synthetic fiber that takes moisture away from your feet faster than cotton. Wear shower shoes when using public showers.

Other Common Foot Ailments

PLANTAR WARTS

Description: may appear on the soles of the feet and are caused by a virus. They may be related to stress which increases the susceptibility to the virus. They grow deep into the skin, usually this growth occurs slowly. There are two types of plantar warts. A *solitary wart* – a single wart that often increases in size and *mosaic warts* – which are a cluster of several small warts growing closely together in one area.

Symptoms: include thickened skin (similar to calluses), pain when walking or standing, and tiny black dots may often appear on the surface of the warts.

Causes: Plantar Warts can be contagious and frequently family members may develop them. If someone in your family has developed a wart or warts, make sure they use their own bath mat and towel, since wet, porous surfaces may contain the virus. The bathtub or the shower stall bottom itself, which is nonporous, will probably not harbor the virus.

Treatment: Adequate intake of Vitamin C & CoQ10 daily is important to maintain immunity against viruses that cause warts.

Try these at-home remedies: apply fresh, peeled garlic directly to the wart. Cover it with duct tape to let the garlic target the wart, and then remove. Apply new garlic every day, avoiding contact with healthy surrounding skin. Or you can try a compress or cotton ball soaked in vinegar and tape it down on the wart with an elastic bandage for at least one or two hours daily. Vitamin E oil is also said to work against warts. Once a day, pierce a vitamin E capsule and rub the contents into the wart.

Warts may disappear on their own. Don't attempt to burn or cut off warts yourself. If, after reasonable time, they don't disappear, further diagnostic evaluation may be necessary. See your foot doctor for treatment or to rule out other potential causes for the growth. Unless warts become bothersome, sore or interfere with walking, there is no need to see a doctor.

RASHES

Description: a noticeable change in the texture or color of the skin. When you notice a rash, it's important that you get to the bottom of what type it is so you can treat it effectively.

Symptoms: Skin may become itchy, bumpy, chapped, scaly or otherwise irritated.

Causes: Rashes are caused by a wide range of conditions including: Athlete's Foot, poison ivy, eczema, shoe contact dermatitis, allergies, medication and cosmetics.

Treatment: If you suspect *poison ivy* – an itchy, blistering rash that begins 12-72 hours after coming into contact with the oil from the plant – apply a cold compress to the rash. Also use a skin protectant like baking soda and oatmeal to dry out the rash, relieve minor irritation and itching and to stop oozing.

Eczema: Dyshidrotic eczema is a common form of eczema that affects the soles of the feet. Dyschidrotic eczema has some unique features, including: painful and itchy deep-set blisters on the soles of the feet; redness; flaking; and scaly, cracked skin. Treatment for dyshidrotic eczema can include soaking the feet in cool water several times a day before applying a rich moisturizer or skin barrier repair cream. You can also use a cold compress to cool the affected area.

Shoe Contact Dermatitis: is a rash caused by an allergic reaction to your shoes or socks. It is generally an itchy and peeling rash on the balls of the feet, bottom of the toes, or heels. The rash bumps may also blister. If you have an allergic reaction to your shoes, the first step of treatment will be to minimize contact to the allergen. The reaction will typically clear up on its own. A cool compress can make you feel more comfortable from the itching.

In general do not scratch your rash. Use apple cider vinegar and water (50/50 mix) and spray on effected areas to help soothe the itch. You can also use a cold compress to cool the affected area.

199

Laughter is inner jogging, good for your body and soul. – Norman Cousins

Rash information from web: www.verywellhealth.com

Body Misalignment Can Cause Foot Problems

If you suffer from foot disorders and pain it would be a good idea to consult a Chiropractor, who is experienced in the relief of pain, and the correction of skeletal and connecting tissue misalignments. Everyone is at risk of suffering foot trouble, however, particularly susceptible are diabetics, athletes, dancers, those who are overweight and older citizens.

Chiropractic, which is derived from the Greek words 'chiros' and 'praktikos' which mean 'done by hand', looks at the relationship between the spinal column, the skeletal system and the connecting soft tissue and nerves in the restoration and maintenance of health. It was developed by a Canadian, Dr. Daniel David Palmer in Davenport, Iowa who performed the first chiropractic adjustment on September 18, 1885. However, cruder forms of physical manipulation had been practiced for thousands of years in ancient Greece, Rome, India and the Orient. Even Hippocrates, the father of modern medicine used such methods of healing way back in 400 B.C. (For more information on Chiropractic see page 231).

ART® – A Non-invasive Treatment

ART® stands for Active Release Techniques®. It is a highly successful hands-on treatment method to address the problems in the soft tissue of the body, including muscles, ligaments, fascia, and nerves. ART® treatment is highly successful in dealing with foot and ankle injuries because it is specifically designed to locate and treat scar-tissue adhesions that accumulate in the muscles and surrounding soft tissues. Locating and treating the soft-tissue adhesions with ART® allows the practitioner to break up restrictive adhesions, reinstate normal tissue flexibility and movement, and more completely restore flexibility, balance, and stability to the injured area and to the entire kinetic chain.

An additional benefit of ART® is that it allows us to further assess and correct problems not only at the site of pain, but also in other areas of the kinetic chain, which are associated with movement compensations and are often contributing factors to the problem. This ensures that all soft tissue that has become dysfunctional and is contributing to the specific injury is addressed, even if pain has not developed yet. One of the best things about ART® is how quickly it provides results. In our experience, foot injuries respond very well to ART® treatment, especially when combined with appropriate home-stretching exercises. – See: *Activerelease.com*

It's very common during a lifetime, that one will experience a strain or sprain of the foot or ankle. Over time soft tissues may heal, however bones may remain misaligned. Discomfort and complications may continue and could be contributed to a misalignment. Often after one body trauma has been experienced, others follow. This is probably for the same reason.

Treating pain with pain killers is not the right solution. Finding out the root cause of the problem is wiser and more effective! This is where a Chiropractor comes in to examine and if needed, take an x-ray and determine the best course of treatment. Chiropractic foot adjustments can help bring pain relief and restore function. They can prevent problems from spreading from the feet to the knees, hips, entire back, neck and other body areas. For an overview of chiropractic treatment options for a wide range of leg, hip and foot ailments see: *cpsnovi.com/foot-pain/*

Chiropractic Solutions for Foot Problems

The feet are extremely susceptible to many disorders. Feet are complex machines, containing 26 bones, 33 movable joints and a host of ligaments, nerves and blood vessels. They bear the constant weight of our bodies and have to withstand the constant abuse dealt to them daily through walking, standing and running.

Perhaps the most common type of injury is the ankle sprain, but the range of problems threatening the feet is wide, running from a simple stubbed toe or blister to a torn ligament or fracture. Foot pain can arise from badly fitting footwear, from bad walking habits such as favoring one foot over the other, from unevenly distributing body weight as well as from sports injuries.

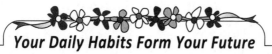

Your Daily Habits Form Your Future

Habits can be wrong or right, good or bad, healthy or unhealthy, rewarding or unrewarding. The right or wrong habits, decisions, actions, words or deeds . . . are up to you! Wisely choose your habits, as they can make or break your life! – Patricia Bragg, Health Crusader

Maintain a healthy, normal weight to avoid strain on your joints and back.

In the same way that foot problems may originate in other body parts, disorders may cause a chain reaction of dysfunctions throughout the body. When you modify your gait and posture due to foot misalignment or malfunction your body may be forced to try and overcompensate, leading to a variety of knee, hip, back and shoulder problems, even to painful headaches.

Walking Promotes Healthy, Happy Feet

There is nothing as pleasurable as walking, it's the most ideal exercise in the world. When taking a walk, open wide your eyes, mind, heart and soul to discover the miracles around you! You will see new beauty in trees, blooming flowers, or singing birds. The seasons of Mother Nature are so rewarding to watch, because each has its own individual beauty!

If you have *feet that are killing you*, all these joys of walking are gone. Many people forego the pleasure of walking because their feet cry out in pain with every step. So, use this *Bragg Foot Care Program* to find new joy in taking healthy walks. Dancing is also a pleasure we enjoy and can and should be pain-free. There is nothing that can relax us more and give us the abandoned joy of living as much as dancing does. But, like walking for pleasure, dancing requires strong, happy feet! These great pleasures in life require pain-free, healthy feet. You can win back youthful feeling feet by being determined to never miss a day in following this foot care program.

The Body is The Hero

It is the body that is the hero, not science, not antibiotics . . . not machines, drugs or new devices. The task of the physician today is what it has always been, to help the body do what it has learned so well to do on its own during its unending struggle for survival to heal itself!"
It is the body, not medicine, that is the hero!
– Ronald J. Glasser, M.D., author *The Body is the Hero*

Wake up and say, "Today I am going to be happier, healthier and wiser in my daily living because I am the captain of my life and in control to steer it for 100% healthy lifestyle living!" Fact: Happy people look younger, live longer, happier and have fewer health problems! – Patricia Bragg

Chapter 19

Your Shoes & Socks Are Very Important

When you cannot go barefoot . . .

Although going barefoot is best for your feet, it is not always possible, or safe, to walk around certain areas without shoes! Sometimes even exercising your feet in the most natural way, out walking barefoot on a beautiful sandy beach or grassy lawn (*hopefully free of toxic chemicals*) at times can be dangerous for many popular beaches are often marred by broken bottles, metal shards, etc. So know areas where you are walking and remember: caution where you step is essential!

It is extremely important to treat your feet to the best shoes available! There are many fine shoes on the market that have been scientifically designed to provide the most natural support for busy, active feet, no matter what they are doing; sitting, walking, standing, jogging, biking, aerobics or competing in a marathon or triathlon!

When looking for healthy shoes, shop at a specialty sports shoe store. These shops sell shoes that are geared for any activity you might wish to undertake, including hiking, tennis and a variety of other sports. Shoes for each of these sports are developed to compensate for any possible stress on different foot parts. For example, the walking shoe is specially cushioned at the heel to protect the foot and the leg from impact at the point of contact with the ground to avoid excess jarring! Hiking shoes or boots are usually steel reinforced around the toe box and ankle to prevent rubbing, stubbing and the possibility of injury from sharp rocks and sticks which are often encountered on hiking trails.

Lucky me, my feet and I love being barefoot. Famous Foot Doctor Scholl said I have the healthiest feet – perfect arches, no blisters, no corns, callouses, aches or pains and I go barefoot most of the time!
– Patricia Bragg

Getting the Proper Shoe Fit

Investing in good, proper fitting shoes will help you keep your feet healthy and happy and will add to your overall feeling of well-being. Remember, your feet carry you through life – so be extra loving and caring to them!

Getting the proper fit is not a hit-or-miss situation. There are basic guidelines you can follow when buying shoes. But the most important rule is this: *If the shoe doesn't feel comfortable, and doesn't provide the support and cushioning you need, please keep looking!*

Don't waste your money and threaten your well-being just because you're in a hurry or because the shoe looks pretty. Plan ahead. Buy shoes well before you need them for a special event, whether it be a party, a big hike or a triathlon. A race could be lost with the wrong new shoes – we have seen it happen when we trained athletes! You may need time to break the shoes in. Haste often makes waste when buying shoes! Plan your shoe needs ahead of time and shop wisely!

The best possible shoe you can buy is one that is lightweight with a flat heel simulating the bare foot. Shoes should be of a natural material that is flexible. Avoid shoes that are made of plastic or other man-made materials. Such shoes most often will not provide the proper foot support. Also feet can't breathe in plastic! The best shoe materials are leather (including suede) or canvas. Leather adapts or molds itself to the shape of your foot and generally lasts a longer time than other materials. Canvas, such as that used in many sports shoes, has the same flexibility. Both materials absorb moisture that helps reduce fungal infections and the discomfort and embarrassment of foot perspiration.

Wear proper fitting footwear at all times as there are over 280 different foot ailments that can be suffered. – American Podiatric Medical Association

---

The world is moving so fast now-a-days that the man who says it can't be done is generally interrupted by someone doing it. – Elbert Hubbard

---

True wisdom consists in not departing from Mother Nature, but molding our conduct according to her Wise Mothering Laws. – Seneca

How to Buy Comfortable, Healthy Shoes

Buy shoes after carefully trying on the shoes that first seem to meet your various uses and needs (sports, casual, work, dress, etc.). Shopping for shoes in the late afternoon or early evening will help you get an accurate fit, as feet tend to be slightly larger after spending the day on them. Also, with age and usually during pregnancy, feet tend to get larger and wider. Most people have one foot larger than the other, so make sure the salesperson measures both feet and fits the shoes to the larger one. *Remember, how your feet feel affects your whole general health, mood, energy and well-being.*

Stand up and walk around the store when trying on shoes. You should have at least a half-inch of space between the end of the shoe and your longest toe while standing with your full weight on your feet. The back of the shoe, however, should fit snugly without any rubbing or slipping up and down that could cause heel blisters. Be sure and wear the right stockings or socks when trying on shoes.

Width as well as length is important in buying shoes. Move your fingers across top of shoe with your foot in it. A ripple of leather should be evident with a proper fit. Avoid shoes that are too tight at the foot's widest point. Buy shoes that are the proper width for your feet.

Check by feeling the inside of both shoes to make sure there are no stitching ridges, wrinkles, bumps, hard seams or any other protrusions that will rub against your feet and cause blisters or other irritations. Flexible shoe soles are desirable – hold shoe upside down and bend between sole and heel area to check for flexibility. *Avoid all pointed shoes or boots that pinch the toes and throw the foot off balance causing corns, bunions, posture problems and many other health problems!*

Check out these popular shoes on their websites:

- www.eccoUSA.com
- www.Asics.com
- www.Rockport.com
- www.thewalkingcompany.com
- www.NewBalance.com
- www.Birkenstock.com

Check out this website for more tips on how to get a proper shoe fit:
www.whentheshoefits.com/pages/proper-fit

Socks of Natural Materials are Best!

Not only shoes, but socks also, should be made of natural materials, either cotton or wool or a blend of the two. Silk, another natural material from which socks are made, can be worn under other socks in extremely cold weather. Socks made of synthetic fabrics don't absorb perspiration and this keeps the feet trapped in moisture. A warm, wet environment is conducive to the growth of bacteria and fungi and is especially to be avoided during strenuous exercise when the feet perspire profusely. Wearing socks made of synthetics, especially when they are worn all day, can result in fungal infections and in cracking and bleeding between toes.

Custom Molded Shoes Are Beneficial

Custom molded shoes are made from an exact plaster cast of your foot. These are particularly beneficial for people who suffer with high insteps, fallen arches or foot genetic problems. Although they are expensive, molded shoes are well constructed with flexible soles and should provide good service for several years with normal use. In most cases, the manufacturer will provide a guarantee that the shoe will survive the usual wear and tear for a certain period of time. Be sure to check on guarantees if you are in the market for a molded shoe. Also, be sure to seek out a reputable manufacturer who takes careful measurements of your feet and makes a working plaster cast. Some better shoes, short of molded shoes and special orthopedic shoes, are the Birkenstock and Ecco brands, which follow the natural foot curve – but be sure the sole is flexible! They come in a wide variety of sandal and shoe styles and most styles will pamper your feet in the most natural way, short of going barefoot. Also, lately in some models, the soles are too stiff which hinders the foot's flexibility.

(206)

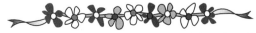

It's magnificent to live long if one keeps healthy, fit, alert, pain-free, youthful and active enjoying a happy, fulfilled life! – Harry Fosdick

There are only two ways to live your life. One is as though nothing is a miracle. The other is as though everything is a miracle. – Albert Einstein

High Heels Can Cause Pain and Wreck Health

Women should wear high heels with caution, and then only for special occasions. Low-heeled shoes are the best choice for day-to-day wear as they keep heels flat to the ground, much like walking barefoot as Mother Nature intended! High heels force the whole body forward, causing the back to curve in, the stomach to protrude and muscles in the legs to shorten. Women's female organs suffer from being tilted and off balance while walking in high heals (*on toes and balls of feet*). This is your body's way of compensating for being thrown off balance, but it can result in mounting aches and pains from your toes to your back and neck.

Tips for Buying the Best Sport Shoes

When you run, your feet hit the ground more than 1,000 times per mile! In aerobics, the weight of your body slams into your soles, which are usually hitting against a concrete or wood-based floor (most gyms have a layer of carpeting down to cushion impact, but unless specially constructed to be spring-loaded the layer under the carpet is generally very hard). Tennis and other racquet sports cause you to twist and turn your feet unnaturally when reaching to return a wayward shot.

So you can see the importance of spending your money to buy a well-made specific sport shoe that is designed especially to be supportive, cushioned in the right places and comfortable for your feet! By wearing the proper sports footwear, you reduce your chances of developing overuse injuries such as shin splints, arch strain, blisters and tendonitis.

The ideal sport shoe will not only support your feet, but will provide cushioning to the ankles, knees, hips and back! You can also give yourself extra protection by investing in *Dr. Scholl's Air-Pillo® Comfort Insoles* or other foot pads found in local sport stores. You can cut them to fit perfectly inside any shoe. If you use them regularly, be sure and take a pair with you when trying on future new shoes! This is an inexpensive way to provide additional comfort to any shoe, but especially walking, running, sport and dancing shoes.

Sports Shoes Buying Check List

When shopping for sport shoes, use this selection method to make certain you get the best, most comfortable shoes that will fit your body's needs:

- When standing, you should be able to put the width of your index finger between the end of the shoe and your longest toe. This is extremely important, for when the sole hits the ground, the shoe will grab and your foot will slide forward. If the shoes are too short, they will create a jamming, stubbing action on the toes, resulting in sore, swollen toes and can even cause black toenails. (If you have shoes like this, give them to your local thrift store – they might fit someone.)

- While holding the shoe in your hands, flex the sole at the ball of the foot. If the shoe only bends at the arch, there is not enough support, the lack of which could lead to knee pain, a crucial situation for runners and other athletes. The sole should be flexible, yet firm throughout its length.

- Again holding the shoe, squeeze the sides of the heels where they join the sole. This area should be very firm in order to keep your heel supported and eliminate slipping (heel pads are available, if needed). Proper fitting shoes will do away with blisters and calluses, while reducing problems in the ankles, shins and knees.

Composition of Sports Shoes:

- **The Outsole:** This part contacts the ground and takes the most abuse. It should provide traction as well as shock absorption. The waffle-bottom soles are designed for cross-country running because they provide a gripping property and stability in wet grass or dirt. They're not suitable for cement or wood floors.

- **The Midsole:** This is between the outsole and the insole. It is usually a cushioning material such as ethylene vinyl acetate (EVA), which not only provides cushioning, but also stability in a shoe.

- **The Insole:** This is the inner lining of the shoe, usually removable, designed to cushion your foot. Many models come with arch support inserts.

- **Heel Counter:** This is the rigid shoe material that encompasses the heel. Most shoes have an internal heel counter but some have an external heel counter or stabilizer made of hard plastic at the base of the heel counter to help control excessive heel rotation. This is an important part of any quality running shoe.
- **The Upper:** The upper part is no longer limited to leather or canvas. Today, uppers are often made of a combination of materials, including nylon mesh for breathability and pigskin for support.
- **Lacing:** There are many lacing systems available, including speed laces that use hooks instead of eyelets and convenient (*easy to do*) velcro backed strap fasteners.

Here are Shoes for Different Sports:

- **Aerobic Shoes** should be lightweight enough for dance moves, but durable. The outsole needs to be more flexible and a stiff heel counter helps prevent overuse syndromes. Those with weak ankles should consider hightops.
- **Tennis Shoes** tend to be heavier to provide more stable support for the side to side movements required for tennis. Leather uppers are popular for support and durability. A rigid heel counter is again recommended.
- **Basketball Shoes** also need to be heavier than running shoes for additional support and durable enough to withstand the punishment of the sport. The midsole should be firmer than running shoes for more ankle support and provide shock absorption. A stiff heel counter, hightops and cushioned innersoles are all recommended to reduce the chance of ankle injuries.
- **Running Shoes** should have at least a half-inch of midsole cushion to absorb shock and should also have a stiff heel counter. Make sure when fitting that your shoe has a roomy toe box. Allow at least a half-inch extra toe length in all shoes. During runs, the feet can often swell by a full shoe size or more.

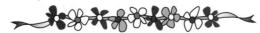

The seat of knowledge is in the head; of wisdom, in the heart.
We are sure to judge wrong if we do not feel right. – William Hazlitt

80% of all foot problems can be attributed to ill-fitting footwear.
– Dr. William A. Rossi, Podiatrist and consultant to the footwear industry

Runners Need Good Shoes

If you are a runner who weighs more than 180 pounds, you should make extra sure you purchase a shoe designed to carry the weight. Most running shoes are designed for the light to mid-weight runner (no more than 175 pounds). The vertical impact on the shoe increases quickly for heavier runners and can lead to more injuries. Ask your sports shoe salesman for shoes specifically designed for heavyweight runners. Also consider adding your own insole (such as *Dr. Scholl's*) to help dissipate the ground impact.

Avoid the temptation to buy cheap running shoes, or to use shoes not designed for running. Sports physicians note that one potential consequence is excessive, repetitive trauma to the sensory nerve passing along the inside of the heel. The nerve sheath begins to enlarge into a heel neuroma and pressure on the nerve fibers produces a mild burning or tingling sensation at first, that later develops into pain. If the runner continues despite the pain, it can lead to constant heel pain that requires surgery. This condition is most likely to occur in people who have excessive pronation.

Many people use running shoes for walking shoes, but serious walkers should purchase a shoe made for walking. The foot operates much differently in walking than in running. There is a smoother heel-toe transition, and the impact on the heel is much less for walkers. A beveled heel is recommended. The outsole should be extremely flexible. Some additional midsole cushioning is built in to propel the walker off the midfoot and onto the ball of the foot. The heel counter doesn't have to be as stiff. Uppers should be breathable with pigskin reinforcement for lateral movement.

Wearing the right shoes for your sport helps guarantee a better performance with pain free feet in the sport and activity of your choice. Remember, take care of your feet and they will take care of you for your entire lifetime!

Women have four times as many foot problems as men do.

Keep your feet happy with comfortable shoes and a proper fit.

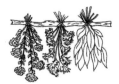

Chapter 20

The Healing Properties of Herbs

*Herbal, Holistic and Dietary Remedies
For Foot and Joint Ailments*

*"You are what you eat, drink, breathe, think,
say and do!"*

"What is on the plate today, we become tomorrow."
– Patricia Bragg

With these two wise Bragg epithets in mind we may deduce that we can address imbalances and dysfunctions within our body by looking at what we put into it. Whereas damage may already have been done due to years of bad dietary habits, the body has incredible recuperative powers if only we give it a chance to use them.

For example, in dietary terms there is a strong direct correspondence between certain foods and beverages and gout. As we know, gout is caused by a build-up of uric acid crystals in the joints of the foot. Certain foods (generally protein rich foods) are high in a compound called purine which raises uric acid levels. Therefore limiting or eliminating altogether the intake of these foods will help lower the frequency and intensity of gout attacks. Cut out red meats, bouillon and gravies, liver, kidney, sweetbreads and other organ meats, coffee, refined sugar and white-flour products, alcohol, spices, shrimp, scallops, anchovies, and rich, greasy and oily foods in general.

What to eat: brown rice, celery, tomatoes, seaweed, cherries, blueberries, bananas, kale, cabbage, parsley and all leafy green vegetables. What to drink: pure water, vegetable and fruit juices – especially cherry, carrot, parsley and celery juice. See herbs pages 213-220 for effective remedies for existing gout and joint symptoms.

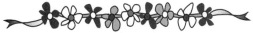

*You cannot have a foot problem without having that problem reflected in
other parts throughout your body. – Dr. Elizabeth H. Roberts, Podiatrist*

Remedies for Athlete's Foot, Foot Odor & Smelly Shoes

For athlete's foot a variety of herbal remedies can be taken both orally and applied to the area of an infection itself. Having some helpings of acidophilus or soy yogurt each day also creates good bacteria which combats the unwanted bad bacteria that causes athlete's foot.

Here are some natural treatments which can be applied directly to athlete's foot: after thoroughly washing the feet with warm soapy water, rinsing and drying, massage in garlic oil 2 to 3 times daily. Onion juice may be applied in the same way until symptoms reduce. Alternatively, soak feet twice daily in a solution of organic apple cider vinegar and 70% warm water. Black walnut tincture is another well tried remedy to be applied externally and frequently until you see improvement.

Finally, try soaking your feet in black tea. Add 2-3 tea bags to a pot of boiling water. Cool mixture, and soak feet for a half-hour. Tannic acid in black tea kills some of the fungus and provides soothing relief for painful feet.

To combat foot odor try this wonderful foot soak: pour two quarts of hot water into a foot bowl and add a half cup of organic apple cider vinegar and 10 drops of tea tree essential oil and mix thoroughly. Soak feet in this solution for 15-30 minutes, and allow to dry in air for at least 5 minutes.

To overcome smelly shoes make mixture of 3 Tbsps. ground dried sage leaves and 3 Tbsps. of baking soda. Sprinkle 1 Tbsp. of mixture into shoes at night, shake around entire inside of shoes and leave overnight. Wear shoes the following day with mixture still inside, and remove and replace with fresh mixture nightly.

SAGE

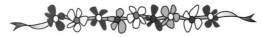

The first wealth is your health. – Ralph Waldo Emerson

 Healthy organic foods and herbs have an abundance of potential life energy!

Herbs and Their Healing Properties to Relieve Foot Ailments, Gout and Arthritis

Mother Nature has strewn the earth with a myriad of plants and herbs with miraculous, but often underestimated healing powers, yet still mankind has chosen to go down the road of creating artificial chemicals to try and cure his ills. It's important to understand that we are part of nature, and that our own natural pharmacy is all around us in nature, forests and oceans.

African Ginger (Zingiber Officinale). Ginger has been used in Chinese medicine for over 2,500 years for ailments ranging from diarrhea to rheumatism. In the Ayurvedic healing tradition it is used for treating inflammatory joint diseases such as arthritis. It is the underground stem, or rhizome, that is used, usually in powder form. The usual dosage is 2-4 grams, 2-3 times daily. Also slices of fresh ginger root may be steeped in boiling water and the liquid applied as a poultice on a flannel cloth, applied directly to arthritic areas, as warm as the body can bear, to help relieve discomfort.

Birch Leaf (Betula Alba). An infusion of Birch Leaf can be prepared for flushing out uric acid from joints and for alleviating arthritic pain. Add 1 Tbsp. fresh leaves to $^{1}/_{2}$ cup of boiling water. Cool, and take twice per day.

Boswellia (Boswellia Serrata). This is a resin gleaned from a tree which proliferates in India. Many studies have shown that Boswellia is potent in the treatment of osteoarthritis and rheumatoid arthritis. About 150 mgs. three times daily of the standardized extract of the gum oleoresin of Boswellia is the usual dosage. It is recommended you continue this for 8 to 12 weeks.

Briar Hip & Blueberry (Rosa Canina, Vaccinium Myrtillus). All the berries in the blue/black family have potent diuretic properties and flush out uric acid from joints.

Superfoods (fruits, vegetables, grains, nuts and seeds) are foods found in nature. They are superior sources of anti-oxidants and essential nutrients and have been proven to help prevent and even reverse cardiovascular disease, Type 2 Diabetes, hypertension and certain cancers.

Buchu (Barosma Betulina). A Buchu herbal infusion may be taken 3 times per day, adding one teaspoon of the fresh leaves (2 tsps. if dried leaves are used) to a cup of boiling water, allowing to brew for a good 5 minutes, then strain. This bush, a native of South Africa, has been used to treat so many ailments that it has been described by medical botanists as being *'the Buchu plant used to treat every disease which afflicts mankind.'*

Burdock (Arctium Lappa). Burdock is a biennial plant found near fences and roadsides. The root of Burdock is effective in the treatment of gout and rheumatism. In Japan, the roots and leaf stalks are boiled twice then eaten. In the west the traditional dosage is 2-4 ml of burdock root tincture per day. For the dried root in capsule form, 1-2 grams may be taken three times per day.

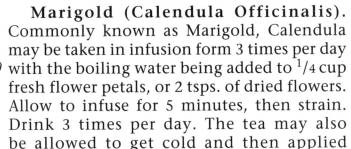

Marigold (Calendula Officinalis). Commonly known as Marigold, Calendula may be taken in infusion form 3 times per day with the boiling water being added to $^1/4$ cup fresh flower petals, or 2 tsps. of dried flowers. Allow to infuse for 5 minutes, then strain. Drink 3 times per day. The tea may also be allowed to get cold and then applied directly to infected area using a soft cloth. This flower with anti-fungal and antibacterial properties has been used to treat other skin ailments such as eczema and skin ulcerations. The flowers have been used as a food coloring and for flavoring soups, vegetables and salads.

Marigold

Cayenne (Capsicum Frutescens). Cayenne contains a resinous substance known as Capsaicin which provides pain relief by acting on sensory nerves. The effect is temporary, but effective, in providing relief from arthritic pain. It is the fruit that proffers the capsaicin, which is normally administered in cream form. Its counter-irritant action – diverting attention from the original source of pain by depleting neurotransmitters sent out by nerves to the problem area – lends its potency in treating joint pain. Cayenne is usually applied in cream form, although an infusion can be prepared using

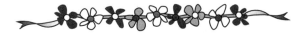

Everything in excess is opposed by nature. – Hippocrates

^{1}/2 to 1 tsp. of powder to a cup of boiling water. To keep your feet warm sprinkle 2 Tbsps. of cayenne pepper into a pair of woolen socks. Put on a pair of white cotton socks, and over these the woolen socks with the cayenne pepper. Your feet will stay warm and toasty.

Celery (Apium Graveolens). Both the crushed seeds and the juice of the celery (stalks, leaves) plant are potent in the treatment of rheumatoid arthritis and gout due to their diuretic properties. To make an infusion, pour a cup of boiling water over 1-2 tsps. of freshly crushed seeds and let stand for 10-15 minutes. Take 3 times per day. For juice, use a juicer to extract fresh juice. Take 1-2 Tbsps. 2 or 3 times per day one hour before meals.

Cherry (Prunus Serotina). Having organic cherry concentrated juice, dried cherries or eating a ^{1}/2 pound of cherries on a daily basis has proven effective in the lowering of uric acid levels and the prevention of gout attacks. Cherries are rich in anthocyanidins (flavonoids with anti-inflammatory properties), which also help to neutralize excess acidity – in particular uric acid.

Clove (Caryophyllus Aromaticus). In Chinese medicine cloves have long been used to treat athlete's foot and other fungal infections, and medieval German herbalists used them as a gout treatment. Cloves have antimicrobial properties effective against fungi and bacteria. Apply cotton wool dipped in clove oil to the affected area. Or prepare an infusion of 1 tsp. clove powder to 1 cup of boiling water. Drink 3 times per day.

Coix (Coicis Lachryma-jobi). Also known as Job's Tears, the seeds of this herb may be used to treat rheumatic and arthritic symptoms. To infuse add 1-3 ounces to a cup of boiling water. Alternatively prepare a porridge of 3 grams of Coix and Cinnamon-twig tea with brown rice.

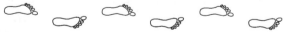

Follow the steps of the Godly instead, and stay on the right path,
for good men enjoy life to the full. – Proverbs 2:20-21

Wear proper fitting footwear at all times as there are over 280 different
foot ailments that can be suffered. – American Podiatric Medical Assoc.

Follow Mother Nature and God – the rewards are great! – Patricia Bragg

Comfrey (Symphytum Officinale). For an effective treatment to reduce pain and inflammation during pronounced arthritic attacks, make a sap of 1 tsp. comfrey powder or $^1/_3$ tsp. tincture to 3 Tbsp. organic apple cider vinegar. Soak cloth or gauze in mixture and apply to needed area of ankle, foot, or any other area of joint or muscle problems. Leave on overnight, repeating for several nights. Wrap area in soaked gauze and then saran wrap and finally a clean, dry cloth. Leave on overnight. Remove upon awakening in the morning. When the pain has reduced somewhat, massage St. John's Wort Oil into the area before going to bed. This simple mixture helps promotes inner healing.

Daisy (Bellis Perennis). The daisy flowers have a reputation for being beneficial against arthritic and rheumatic symptoms. To infuse, pour a cup of boiling water onto 1 tsp. of dried daisies and allow to brew for 10 minutes. Take 3 to 4 times daily.

Evening Primrose (Oenothera Biennis). Evening primrose oil is beneficial for the treatment of rheumatoid arthritis, diabetes and helps relieve menopausal symptoms. The oil contains gamma linolenic acid (GLA) which promotes the production of prostaglandin E1 (PGE1), an important hormone-like substance. Conditions such as diabetes impede the body's natural production of GLA. 3,000-6,000 mgs. of evening primrose oil daily is recommended which provides 270-360 mgs. of GLA.

Gotu Kola (Centella Asiatica). The leaves of this perennial plant native to India, Sri Lanka and other tropical countries have properties which make them an effective herbal combatant of athlete's foot. Prepare an infusion by adding boiling water to $^1/_4$ cup of fresh leaves or 2 tsps. of the dried variety. To annul the bitter taste somewhat you may add honey or lemon. Let stand for 5 minutes, strain and drink. You may also apply as a wet compress bandage, cover with plastic wrap, and then cover foot with a cotton sock.

The civilized man has built a coach, but has lost the use of his feet.
– Ralph Waldo Emerson

Gravel Root (Eupatorium Purpureum). The rhizome and the root may be used to prepare an infusion to treat rheumatoid arthritis and gout. Pour 1 cup of boiling water over 1 tsp. of the fresh herb and allow to infuse for 10 minutes. Drink 3 times per day.

Guaiacum (Guaiacum Officinale). Guaiacum, the resin from a tree native to Central and South America, Mexico and the West Indies, is useful in the treatment of gout and the prevention of its recurrence, also to alleviate symptoms of rheumatoid arthritis. To make an infusion pour boiling water over 1 tsp. of the wood chips and allow to stand for 15 to 20 minutes. You may drink this infusion 3 times per day.

Guggul (Commiphora Mukul). Guggul is a gum resin obtained from a small tree (also known as the Mukul Myrrh Tree), which is native to India and certain Arab countries. The resin is used in Ayurvedic medicine for the treatment of inflammatory conditions such as rheumatoid arthritis and gout. It is normally taken as a herbal supplement in tablet form.

Gymnema (Gymnema Sylvestre). This climbing plant that is found in Central and Southern India has been used for the treatment of diabetes for over 2,000 years. The leaves have the effect of lowering blood sugar and raising insulin levels. 400 mgs. per day for periods of up to 18 or 20 months have been recommended. Alternatively 2 to 4 grams of leaf powder may be used.

Horsetail (Equisetum Arvense). This healing herb is renowned for its usefulness in treating arthritis and gout. An infusion taken 3 times daily will help eliminate uric acid build up. Horsetail contains Potassium, 15 types of bioflavonoids and is rich in silicates. This natural silicon content is the active anti-arthritic agent. Pour boiling water over 2 Tsps. of the dried Horsetail, allowing to infuse for 15 to 20 minutes. $3^1/2$ ounces of Horsetail added to bath water makes a soothing bath to alleviate arthritic pains.

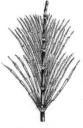

Horsetail

Now learn what and how great benefits of a temperate diet will bring along with it. In the first place, you will enjoy good health. – Horace, 95 B.C.

Kelp (Fucus Vesiculosus). This sea vegetable is also known as Bladderwrack and is reputed to alleviate symptoms of rheumatoid arthritis both by taking internally in infusion form, and using externally, by applying the same topically to inflamed joints. Pour 1 cup boiling water onto 2 tsps. dried (*or powder*) kelp. Take 3 times daily. (*We sprinkle kelp granules over our food.*)

Marsh Clover (Menyanthes Trifoliata). Also known as Bogbean, Bog Myrtle and Marsh Trefoil, the leaves of this herb have diuretic properties and are renowned for their beneficial action against osteoarthritis and rheumatoid arthritis. For an infusion pour a cup of boiling water onto 1-2 tsps. of the dried leaves. Allow to steep for 10-15 minutes. The infusion may be taken 3 times per day.

Parsley (Petroselinum Crispum). An infusion of Parsley can be prepared to help flush out uric acid from tissues and joints and to help alleviate arthritic pain. Pour 1 cup of boiling water on to 1-2 tsps. of fresh leaves or root and infuse for about 5-10 minutes in a closed container. Take twice per day. Parsley should not be used during pregnancy or if you have a kidney infection.

218 Parsley

Sarsaparilla (Ichnocarpus Frutescens). Used widely in Ayurvedic medicine, Sarsaparilla root is excellent for gout, and a poultice of the infusion of the root and leaves may be applied topically to painful, arthritic joints. Pour 1 cup of boiling water over 1 tsp. dried sarsaparilla powder. Drink twice daily or apply direct to affected area.

Stinging Nettle (Urtica Dioica). Drinking a cup of stinging nettle tea 3 times per day for 3 weeks will help eliminate uric acid build up in the joints. Stinging nettles strengthen the whole body, are an excellent general detoxifier and are particularly effective in the treatment of arthritis. Pour boiling water onto 1-3 teaspoons of the dried herb and allow to infuse for 10-15 minutes.

Visit this great informative website on herbs: www.herbs.org

Herbs can be very helpful with stress, sleep disturbances and anxiety.

Tea Tree (Melaleuca Alternifolia). In 1770, Captain James Cook came across a grove of trees with aromatic leaves from which he and his party made tea. It was not until much later (after the first world war) that the real medicinal properties of Tea Tree Oil were investigated. Among the essential oils, tea tree has few rivals with regards to its anti-infectious properties. It was discovered that the oil of the tea tree is 12 times stronger than carbolic acid as an antiseptic bactericide. Tea tree is powerfully antibiotic and extremely beneficial to the human body and immune system. Tea tree oil is potent in the treatment and prevention of a number of bacterial, viral and fungal infections.

To treat Athlete's foot, apply a few drops of the oil to the infected area 4 times per day until it appears that the problem has cleared. Continue to apply for two to four weeks afterwards to make sure every trace of the fungi has disappeared.

Turmeric (Curcuma Longa). Turmeric's anti-inflammatory properties make it potent in treating arthritis. Recommended dose is 400 mgs. 3 times daily.

White Poplar (Populus Tremuloides). This herb has the reputation of being effective in the treatment of rheumatoid arthritis, especially in reducing discomfort when there is much pain and swelling. May also be used for arthritis in conjunction with other herbs such as celery, bogbean and black cohosh. Put 1-2 tsps. of the dried bark in a cup of water, bring to a boil and allow to infuse for 10-15 minutes. May be drunk 3 times per day.

Wild Yam (Dioscorea Villosa). The dried roots of this herb are excellent for the treatment of rheumatoid arthritis, especially for soothing and subduing acute periods of intense inflammation. Put 1-2 tsps. of the dried root into a cup of water, bring to a boil and allow to simmer for 10-15 minutes. Should be taken 3 times per day.

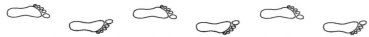

Lavender helps you relax. Before drying off in the shower, place 3 drops of essential lavender oil on a damp sponge or washcloth and gently rub it over your body. The soothing, relaxing active agents in the lavender oil will enter your body through your skin and nose.

Willow (Salix Alba). The bark from this tree native to central and southern Europe and North America has analgesic, anti-inflammatory and pain relieving qualities, which prove effective in the treatment of osteoarthritis and rheumatoid arthritis. An infusion can be prepared by boiling 1-2 grams of bark in 200 ml of water for 10 minutes. This can be drunk up to 5 times per day.

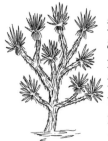

Yucca (Yucca Schidigera). This desert tree is useful for the treatment of osteoarthritis and rheumatoid arthritis. A study has revealed that saponins (soapy textured fluids) from the yucca stop the release of toxins from the intestines, which prevent regular formation of cartilage. For arthritis it is recommended to take 2 capsules of yucca twice per day on an empty stomach.

It's Important To Remember The Following When Using Herbal Remedies:

Pregnant women and diabetics should consult an herb specialist or their health doctor before embarking on a course of herbal therapy. It's also important to take into consideration that some herbs when taken alongside conventional prescription medication may cause adverse reactions - again advice should be sought.

For more herbal info visit these websites:

- *www.NaturalHerbsGuide.com*
- *www.herbs.org*
- *www.LaceToLeather.com/SafeNaturalCures.html*

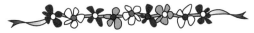

Herbs can be taken in a variety of healthy forms, including tinctures, tonics, salves, oils and teas.

"Pounding fragrant things – particularly garlic, basil, parsley – is a tremendous antidote to depression. But it applies also to juniper berries, coriander seeds and the grilled fruits of the chili pepper. Pounding these things produces an alteration in one's being – from sighing with fatigue to inhaling with pleasure. The cheering effects of herbs and alliums cannot be too often reiterated. Virgil's appetite was probably improved equally by pounding garlic as by eating it." – Patience Gray

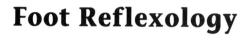

Chapter 21

Foot Reflexology

Foot reflexology is a form of therapy that involves manipulating specific areas, or zones of the body. These zones are directly linked to the reflex points of all of the various organs and nerves in the body. The most sensitive zones are found in the toes, soles, arches and ankles of the feet.

Foot reflexology is an effective way to energize and rebalance the corresponding organs. It is also extremely beneficial in the reduction and even the elimination of pain in the body. In addition, it relieves nervous tension, slows the ageing process, increases circulation and can help you free yourself from illness.

Sound like a miracle? It is! It is a miracle that you can easily learn and use to promote a more healthful, vital way of living for yourself, your family and friends. Everyone, from infants to older people, can benefit from this simple reflexology technique. The accompanying charts are provided to help you learn the basic reflex points. For more info, see: *www.reflexology-usa.net*.

We are proud that Eunice D. Ingham, a pioneer in the reflexology field in America, was a Bragg follower. She became a student during a Bragg Health Crusade in Florida as a young lady and was a faithful follower of our Bragg Healthy Lifestyle all her life. In fact, she said Paul Bragg led her to the study of foot reflexology to help her grandmother's aching feet.

How Does Reflexology Work?

Running between each organ, nerve and gland are channels or currents which send vitalizing energy through our bodies in much the same way that electrical wires carry electrical currents. Often, a channel becomes blocked because of illness, injury or nervous tension. Through reflexology and massage, we can open up these blockages and allow the energy to flow freely again.

For example, a winter cold may produce symptoms such as a headache, sore throat, earache and even a stiff neck. By applying pressure to the corresponding zones on the feet in a systematic way, you will be able to relieve these painful and irritating symptoms. This will work whether the problem is a cold, congestion, backache, digestive ailment, poor circulation, insomnia or depression.

Reflexology is Effective Self-Therapy:

1. The feet are easily accessible for reflexologists and great for self-reflexology and massage treatments.

2. The pressure points are simple to find since the feet are tender from being covered and encased most of the time in socks and shoes. In addition, there is little fat or muscle in the feet to interfere with therapeutic effects of massage. It's also possible to feel the buildup of toxic crystal deposits which indicate problems in corresponding body areas.

3. A short cut to learning reflexology is looking at charts that show which body parts correspond to certain areas of the feet. This eliminates the need for advanced anatomy studies.

4. The miracle feet are literally and symbolically our connection with the earth. Because of this, they are especially receptive to the energy which carries us forward each day, and to enhancing that energy.

5. We know that happy pain-free feet are healthy feet. In order to take us through a lifetime, it's important to pamper and protect our feet. Reflexology and foot massages also help improve your general health.

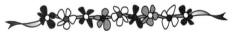

The nation badly needs to go on a healthy diet. It should do something drastic about excessive, unattractive, life-threatening fat. It should get rid of it in the quickest, safest possible way and this is by fasting, exercise and living a healthy lifestyle. – Allan Cott, M.D., author, "Fasting As a Way of Life"

Recent studies revealed that fat stored in the body's "spare tire" around the waist increases risk for diabetes, heart disease and other serious health problems! Shocking fact: the bigger the waistline, the shorter the lifespan!

Reflexology – Pressure Points of the Foot*

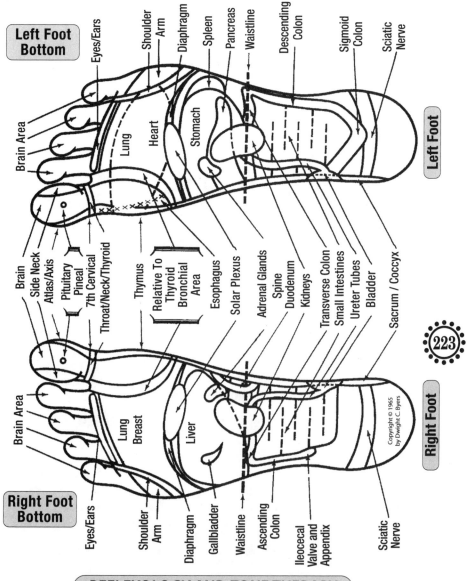

Left Foot Bottom

Eyes/Ears · Shoulder · Arm · Diaphragm · Spleen · Pancreas · Waistline · Descending Colon · Sigmoid Colon · Sciatic Nerve

Brain Area · Lung · Heart · Stomach

Left Foot

Brain · Side Neck · Atlas/Axis · Pituitary · Pineal · 7th Cervical · Throat/Neck/Thyroid · Thymus · Relative To Thyroid Bronchial Area · Esophagus · Solar Plexus · Adrenal Glands · Spine · Duodenum · Kidneys · Transverse Colon · Small Intestines · Ureter Tubes · Bladder · Sacrum / Coccyx

223

Copyright © 1965 by Dwight C. Byers

Right Foot

Brain Area · Lung · Breast · Liver

Right Foot Bottom

Eyes/Ears · Shoulder · Arm · Diaphragm · Gallbladder · Waistline · Ascending Colon · Ileocecal Valve and Appendix · Sciatic Nerve

REFLEXOLOGY AND ZONE THERAPY

Founded by Eunice Ingham, author of "The Story The Feet Can Tell," who was inspired by a Bragg Health Crusade when she was 17. Reflexology helps the body by removing crystalline deposits from meridians (nerve endings) of the feet through deep pressure massage. It helps activate the body's flow of healthy energy by dislodging any collected deposits around the nerve endings. (Charts are reprinted with permission by Eunice Ingham's nephew Dwight Byers). – Visit their website: www.reflexology-usa.net

Reflexology – Pressure Points of the Foot*

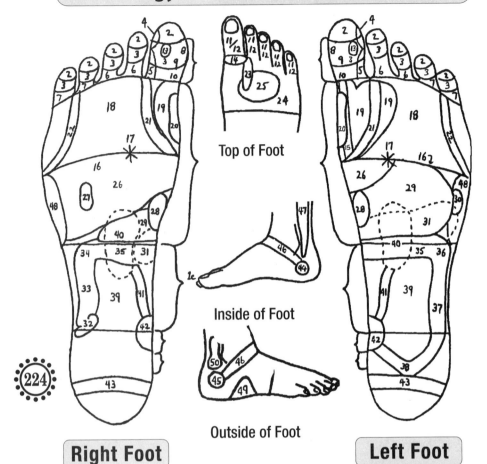

Top of Foot

Inside of Foot

Outside of Foot

224

Right Foot

Left Foot

1. Spine a. Cervical;
   b. Thoracic; c. Lumbar;
   d. Sacrum; e. Coccyx
2. Brain
3. Sinuses
4. Temple
5. Side of Neck
6. Eye, Inner Ear
7. Outer Ear
8. Nose
9. Mouth
10. Throat, Thyroid
11. Jaw (top)
12. Teeth / Gums, (top)
13. Pituitary / Pineal
14. Thyroid / (top), Throat
16. Diaphragm
17. Solar Plexus

18. Lung
19. Heart
20. Thymus
21. Bronchial Tube
22. Shoulder
23. Lymph Drain (top)
24. Ribs / Upper Back (top)
25. Breast / Mammary
    Glands (top)
26. Liver
27. Gallbladder
28. Adrenal
29. Stomach
30. Spleen
31. Pancreas (dotted line)
32. Ileocecal Valve
    (Appendix)
33. Ascending Colon

34. Hepatic Flexure
35. Transverse Colon
36. Splenic Flexure
37. Descending Colon
38. Sigmoid Colon / Flexure
39. Small Intestines
40. Kidney (dotted line)
41. Ureter Tube
42. Bladder / Sacroiliac Joint
43. Sciatic
44. Uterus / Prostate
45. Ovary / Testicle
46. Fallopian Tube /
    Lymph Drain
47. Chronic Area
48. Arm / Hand
49. Hip / Knee / Leg
50. Hip / Sciatic

* Reflexology Center of Honolulu, Hawaii, Reprinted with permission by Jane Kerns

Reflexology – Pressure Points of the Hand

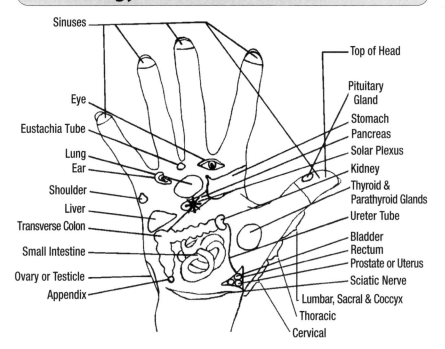

Sinuses

Top of Head

Eye

Pituitary Gland

Eustachia Tube

Stomach
Pancreas

Lung
Ear

Solar Plexus

Kidney

Shoulder

Thyroid & Parathyroid Glands

Liver

Ureter Tube

Transverse Colon

Bladder
Rectum

Small Intestine

Prostate or Uterus

Ovary or Testicle

Sciatic Nerve

Appendix

Lumbar, Sacral & Coccyx
Thoracic
Cervical

How to Perform a Hand Reflexology Massage (on Yourself or Someone Else)

Here are basic steps to doing a hand reflexology massage.

1. Make sure to wash your hands to avoid skin irritations or transfer of infections.

   • Use massage oils or lotion for easier and smoother manipulation of the fingers and hands.

   • Use consistent pressure in a circular motion for 3 to 5 seconds before moving to another area.

   • Refer to the reflexology hand chart for reference to the body part or area you would like to focus on.

2. Start by rubbing your thumb on your palm in wide circles starting from the center of the palm and working your way to the edges. Using a straight motion, rub your thumb pad starting from the knuckles all the way to the wrist. Use light pressure as this move is to help you relax.

3. Grasp a finger and rotate at the joint in a counter-clockwise motion. Do this for all the fingers.

4. Activate your hand pressure points by pressing the ends of each finger between a thumb and forefinger.

5. With your thumb and forefinger, rub counter-clockwise circles starting at the base of each finger all the way to the tip.

6. Use gentle pressure to rub all over the palm, the pads of the fingers, and the back of the hand working your way down to the wrist.

7. Drink water after each hand reflexology session to aid in expelling the wastes and toxins in your system.

Taken from: *mindbodypal.com/hand-reflexology*

Healing Through Reflexology

Reflexologists worldwide have thousands of case histories which testify to the many miraculous healing capabilities of these forms of massage. Although reflexology is not considered a cure for such conditions as terminal illness, broken bones or certain neurological diseases, it has proven extremely effective in treating some health problems and even emotional disorders and infertility. See: *DrLWilson.com/articles/reflexology.htm*

It would be impossible to describe here in detail all the benefits to be derived from this type of therapy. If you are considering using foot reflexology as a healing technique, we recommend you read as many books on the subject as you can find. There are also courses available through community colleges and specialized massage schools which will provide the licensing necessary to practice this art as a professional.

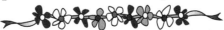

The act of massaging or any form of touch treatment triggers secretion of a natural anti-depressant called serotonin. You can feel this immediately after a therapy session, you're calmer, more focused and suffice to say happier.

Reflexology helps you relax and promotes harmony & balance in your body.

Massage calms the nervous system, allowing better communications between the organs and the body to operate more effectively!

Ten reasons to try Reflexology: relaxation; improved well-being; stress relief; eases tension; improves circulation; detoxes the body; boosts the immune system; helps you sleep; increases energy; speeds up healing.

Setting the Stage For Massage

There is no question that massage, foot reflexology and acupressure (mentioned in the Back Fitness Section pages 118-119) will help promote general well-being and the recovery of sick organs and glands in a safe and more natural way. It's also the most relaxing and caring treatment you can do for someone, including yourself and even pets.

Knowledge of the reflex points is of vital importance. Also, an understanding of the basic strokes and techniques used will make massage a positive and enjoyable experience for both parties involved – the person giving the massage and the recipient. The beauty of massage and foot reflexology is that the more you learn and understand, the greater the health benefits become. Not only will you be helping others, you will be increasing your personal fulfillment through sharing your talent. The act of sharing and giving is its own reward.

A good way to familiarize yourself with reflex points and techniques is to start on your own feet. One rule to remember is to keep the first foot reflexology and massage treatments to about 20 minutes, as the immediate effect of ridding clogged channels of toxins may cause a reaction, such as slight feelings of wooziness or nausea. Begin with a short session, wait one day and then work the feet again.

Relaxation is The Key For Best Treatment

The first step in self foot reflexology is to find the most comfortable, relaxing position to work in. If you are working on your feet, try sitting in a chair, your bed or even on the floor. The location does not matter; the important thing is that you find a comfortable sitting or resting position which permits you to rest the foot you will be massaging on the opposite thigh.

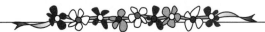

We love helping people who want to live and follow *The Bragg Healthy Lifestyle*! We want to help you now!

When working on someone else's feet, have them lie down or sit in a chair opposite you and rest the foot being treated in your lap. Some reflexologists find it very soothing to have their patients soak the other foot in a basin of warm vinegar-water to stimulate circulation.

The key to successful foot reflexology is relaxation of both the practitioner and the patient. If you are tense or feeling ill, it would be best to postpone the treatment if possible, because your tension will be transferred to the patient's body and you can actually draw energy away from the other person. That will reduce, if not eliminate, the benefits of the treatment. If necessary, get into a relaxed mood with a calming backdrop of candles, flowers and soft music. Environmental sounds, such as ocean waves, waterfalls and singing birds, etc., can be very calming!

If you find you must talk at any time, perhaps to explain what you are doing, speak in soft, hushed tones to maintain the relaxing peaceful mood. Another wonderful way to relax your patient is to wash the feet prior to starting the massage. Many civilizations have used this as a way of welcoming and honoring guests. The host would perform this ritual to show respect and also to soothe the spiritual energy of arriving friends.

Soak the feet for 10 to 15 minutes in warm vinegar-water. It can be plain water, or enhanced with herbal tea bags and a few drops of scented massage oil such as clove, cinnamon or peppermint. Brush the feet vigorously with a cloth or a loofah sponge while feet are still in the water. Dry thoroughly and then start your massage. The feet will be invigorated and sensitive at this point and your patient will be fully relaxed to enjoy maximum pleasure and benefit from the foot and ankle massage treatment.

Make sure your hands are warm before placing them on the feet. This can be done by rubbing them briskly or holding them under warm water. (You should always wash your hands before and after giving a foot and also a body massage for obvious hygienic reasons.)

God has a more acceptable plan. He has a plan to bless you, a plan to heal you, and a plan to protect you!

Be gentle when you first make contact with the feet. This is extremely important for you in order to get a feeling for the overall attitude of the person you massage. Are they tense or relaxed? The initial gentleness will also serve to make the recipient feel more comfortable about you working on their feet. If the person seems tense, just hold one foot for a minute or so to gain their confidence. Then start with a slow, light stroking to get the blood flowing.

Gradually work your way along the sole, over and in between the toes, up the sides of the foot and around to the heels and ankles. Ask the person to tell you if any areas seem more sensitive than others. By studying foot charts, you will be able to pinpoint and pay extra attention to any sensitive problem areas.

A Variety of Massage Techniques to Use

Here are some different massage techniques and strokes you can use to open up blocked channels and encourage the new flow of rejuvenating energy:

- **Kneading** – This is just like working bread dough and can be used to work on large areas of the foot, such as the under-arch. It is very powerful as a means of stimulating muscle reflex points.

- **Vibration** – Put one finger or the heel of the hand on a specific point and move it back and forth in a rapid, gentle motion and then move on to other points. This creates an immediate energy surge to the corresponding organ, nerve or gland.

- **Acupressure** – Use the thumb or knuckle to apply steady and firm pressure to a specific reflex point. Acupressure is excellent for overall toning and for the repairing of corresponding organs.

Self discipline is your golden key;
without it, you can't be happy and healthy.
– Maxwell Maltz, M.D., author "Psycho-Cybernetics"

When your body is completely relaxed then you will experience
an inner peace, inner serenity and the true joy of living.

- **Basic Massage** – Using all the fingers and the thumbs, work quickly and lightly with a release/grip/release/stroke/release/grip action. The result will be very relaxing, yet energizing.

- **Rubbing** – Just as it implies, you rub the feet between your two hands to stimulate blood flow throughout the feet and the entire body.

- **Wringing** – Imagine you are wringing out a wet washcloth, using both hands, twist each hand in opposite directions, going up and down the foot. This motion is one of the most relaxing so it is advisable to have your patient rest after their treatment.

You will, as you study and practice foot reflexology, add other strokes. Some are in books you can read on the subject. Others you will discover for yourself. When you try a new technique, a simple way to gauge its effectiveness is to ask the person you are massaging if it feels good. If so, keep it in your routine.

Each person has a different "pain threshold." That is, some may be able to take a strong, steady pressure to a specific area, say the tips of the toes. Yet another may find it unbearable to have you touch the feet with anything other than a gentle rubbing stroke. Assure your recipient that you will honor their request for harder or softer pressure. If they have this sense of trust in you they will receive greater benefit from the foot treatment.

Foot reflexology is a wonderful, natural way to improve the body's functions and increase your overall health and happiness. It's an art that is easily learned.

The study of foot reflexology will provide you with a method of massage you can share with others, and what greater gift is there than the gift of self? It's a special talent that will add to your joy of living. This alone will make you a happier and more fulfilled person.

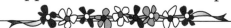

Now, stop and think! Our Creator presented you with the world's most miraculous machine – your own body! This incredible factory has its own non-stop motor (heart), its own fueling system (digestive system), its own filtration system (kidneys), its own thinking computer (brain and nervous system), its own temperature controls (sweat glands), etc. Indeed, this miraculous creation even has the power to reproduce itself!

Chapter 22

Healthy Alternative Therapies
and Massage Techniques

Try Them – They Are Working Miracles!

Explore these wonderful natural methods of healing your body. Finally over 600 Medical Schools in the U.S. are teaching Healthy Alternative Therapies. Please check their websites. Now seek and choose the best healing techniques for you:

ACUPUNCTURE / ACUPRESSURE: Acupuncture directs and rechannels body energy by inserting hair-thin needles (use only disposable needles) at specific points on the body. It's used for pain, backaches, migraines and general health and body dysfunctions. Used in Asia for centuries, acupuncture is safe, virtually painless and has no side effects! Acupressure is based on the same principles and uses finger pressure and massage rather than needles. Check web: *AcupunctureToday.com*

CHIROPRACTIC: was founded in Davenport, Iowa in 1885 by Daniel David Palmer. There are now many schools in the U.S., and graduates are joining Health Practitioners in all nations of the world to share healing techniques. Chiropractic is popular and the largest U.S. healing profession benefitting literally millions! Treatment involves soft tissue, spinal and body adjustment to free your nervous system of any interferences with normal body functions. Its concern is the functional integrity of the musculoskeletal system. In addition to manual methods, chiropractors use physical therapy modalities, exercise, health and nutritional guidance. Web: *ChiroWeb.com*

COLON HYDROTHERAPY: is a safe and effective practice for supporting detoxification, and improving health and vitality. Contact I-ACT (Int'l Association Colon Hydrotherapy) for a certified colon Hydro-Therapist in your area. Web: *i-act.org*

SKIN BRUSHING: daily is wonderful for circulation, toning, cleansing and healing. Use a dry vegetable brush (never nylon) and brush lightly. Helps purify lymph so it's able to detoxify your blood and tissues. Removes old skin cells, uric acid crystals and toxic wastes that come up through skin's pores. Use loofah sponge for variety in shower or tub.

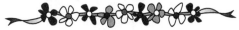

*Skin is often called the 3rd kidney because
it eliminates toxins from the body.*

HOMEOPATHY: In 1796, Dr. Samuel Hahnemann, a German physician, developed homeopathy. Patients are treated with "micro" doses of remedies found in nature to trigger the body's own defenses. This homeopathic principle is a safe and nontoxic remedy and is the #1 alternative therapy in Europe and Britain because it is inexpensive, seldom has any side effects, and usually brings fast results. Web: *HomeopathyCenter.org*

NATUROPATHY: Brought to America by Dr. Benedict Lust, M.D., this treatment uses diet, herbs, homeopathy, fasting, exercise, hydrotherapy, manipulation and sunlight. Practitioners work with your body to restore health naturally. They reject surgery and drugs except as a last resort. Web: *www.Naturopathic.org*

OSTEOPATHY: The first School of Osteopathy was founded in 1892 by Dr. Andrew Taylor Still, M.D. There are now 30 U.S. colleges. Treatment involves soft tissue, spinal and body adjustments that free the nervous system from interferences that can cause illness. Healing by adjustment also includes good nutrition, physical therapies, proper breathing and good posture. Dr. Still's premise: if the body structure is altered or abnormal, then proper body function is altered and can cause pain and illness. Web: *www.AcademyofOsteopathy.org*

232

REFLEXOLOGY/ZONE THERAPY: Founded by Eunice Ingham, author of *Stories The Feet Can Tell*, inspired by a Bragg Health Crusade when she was 17. Reflexology helps the body and organs by removing crystalline deposits from reflex areas (nerve endings) of feet and hands through deep pressure massage. Primitive reflexology originated in China and Egypt and Native American Indians and Kenyans self-practiced it for centuries. Reflexology activates your body's flow of healing and energy by dislodging deposits. Visit Eunice Ingham and nephew Dwight Byer's website: *www.Reflexology-usa.net*

WATER THERAPY: Soothing detox shower: apply organic olive oil to skin, alternate hot and cold water, every 2-3 minutes. Massage body while under hot, filtered spray. Garden hose massage is great in summer or anytime. Hot detox soak bath (diabetics use warm water) 20 minutes with cup of Epsom salts or apple cider vinegar. This soak helps pull out the toxins by creating an artificial fever cleanse.

My father and I want you to enjoy a fulfilled, healthy, long life.
– Patricia Bragg, Pioneer Health Crusader

Time waits for no one, treasure and protect every moment you have!

ALEXANDER TECHNIQUE: helps end improper use of neuromuscular system, helps bring body posture into balance. Eliminates psycho-physical interferences, helps release long-held tension, and aids in re-establishing muscle tone. For more info see web: *AlexanderTechnique.com*

FELDENKRAIS METHOD: Dr. Moshe Feldenkrais founded this in the late 1940s. This Method leads to improved posture and helps create ease and more efficiency of body movement. This Method is a great stress removal. Web: *Feldenkrais.com*

REIKI: A Japanese form of massage that means "Universal Life Energy." Reiki Massage helps the body to detoxify, then re-balance and heal itself. Discovered in the ancient Sutra manuscripts by Dr. Mikao Usui in Japan 1922. Web: *Reiki.org*

ROLFING: Developed by Ida Rolf in the 1930's in the U.S. Rolfing is also called structural processing and postural release, or structural dynamics. It is based on the concept that distortions (accidents, injuries, falls, etc.) and the effects of gravity on the body cause upsets and long-term stress in the body. Rolfing helps to achieve balance and improved body posture. Methods involve the use of stretching, with gentle deep tissue massage and relaxation techniques to loosen old injuries, break bad movement and posture patterns. Web: *Rolf.org*

TRAGERING: Founded by Dr. Milton Trager M.D., who was inspired at age 18 by Paul C. Bragg to become a doctor. It is a mind-body learning method that involves gentle shaking and rocking, allowing the body to let go, releasing tensions and lengthening the muscles for more body peace and health. Tragering can do miracle healing where needed in the body frame, muscles and the entire body. Web: *Trager.com*

MASSAGE & AROMATHERAPY: works two ways: the essence (aroma) relaxes, as does healing massages. Essential oils are extracted from flowers, leaves, roots, seeds and barks. These are usually massaged into skin, inhaled or used in a bath to help the body relax, soothe and heal. The oils, used for centuries to treat numerous ailments, are revitalizing and energizing for the body and mind. Example: Tiger balm, MSM, echinacea and arnica help relieve muscle aches. (Avoid skin creams and lotions with mineral oil – it clogs the skin's pores.) Use these natural oils for the skin: almond, avocado, and I use organic olive oil and mix with aromatic essential oils: rosemary, lavender, rose, jasmine, sandalwood or lemon-balm, etc. – 6 oz. oil and 4 drops of an essential oil. Web: *www.Aromatherapy.com*

MASSAGE – SELF: Paul C. Bragg often said, *"You can be your own best massage therapist, even if you have only one good hand."* Near-miraculous health improvements have been achieved by victims of accidents or strokes in bringing life back to afflicted parts of their own bodies by self-massage and with vibrators. Treatments can be day or night, almost continual. Self-massage also helps achieve relaxation at day's end. Families and friends can learn and exchange massages; it's a wonderful sharing experience. Remember, babies love and thrive with daily massages, start from birth. Family pets also love soothing, healing touch of massages. Web: *RD.com/health/wellness/learn-the-art-of-self-massage*

MASSAGE – SHIATSU: Japanese massage form applies pressure from fingers, hands, elbows and even knees along the same points as acupuncture. Shiatsu originated in Japan and is based on traditional Chinese medicine, and has been widely practiced around the world since 1970s. Shiatsu has been used in Asia for centuries to relieve pain, common ills, muscle stress and to aid lymphatic circulation. See web: *centerpointmn.com/the-benefits-of-shiatsu-massage*

234 *MASSAGE – SWEDISH:* One of the oldest and the most popular and widely used massage techniques. This deep body massage soothes and promotes healthy circulation and is a great way to loosen and relax tight muscles before and after exercise. See web: *www.MassageDen.com/swedish-massage.shtml*

MASSAGE – SPORTS: An important health support system for professional and amateur athletes. Sports massage improves circulation and mobility to injured tissue, enables athletes to recover more rapidly from myofascial injury, reduces muscle soreness and chronic strain patterns. Soft tissues are freed of trigger points and adhesions, thus contributing to improvement of peak neuromuscular functioning and athletic performance.

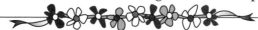

Author's Comment: We have personally sampled many of these Alternative Therapies. It's estimated America's health care costs are over $2.6 trillion. It's more important than ever to be responsible for our own health! This includes seeking dedicated holistic health practitioners to keep us well by inspiring us to practice prevention! These Alternative Healing Therapies are also popular and getting results: aromatherapy, Ayurvedic, biofeedback, guided imagery, herbs, hyperbaric oxygen, music, meditation, magnets, saunas, tai chi, Qi gong, Pilates, Rebounder, yoga, etc. Explore them and be open to improving your earthly temple for a healthy, happier, longer life.

Seek and find the best for your body, mind and soul. – Patricia Bragg

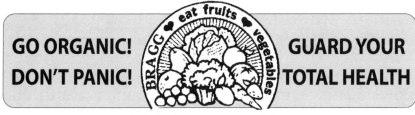

**GO ORGANIC!
DON'T PANIC!**

**GUARD YOUR
TOTAL HEALTH**

FROM THE AUTHORS

This book was written for You! It can be your passport to a healthy, long, vital life. We in the Alternative Health Therapies join hands in one common objective – promoting a high standard of health for everyone. Healthy nutrition points the way – which is Mother Nature and God's Way. This book teaches you how to work with them, not against them! Health doctors, therapists nurses, teachers and caregivers are becoming more dedicated than ever before to keeping their patients healthy and fit. This book was written to emphasize the greatly needed importance of healthy lifestyle living for health and longevity, close to Mother Nature and God.

Statements in this book are scientific health findings, known facts of physiology and biological therapeutics. Paul C. Bragg practiced natural methods of living for over 80 years with highly beneficial results, knowing they were safe and of great value. His daughter Patricia lectured and co-authored Bragg Health Books with him and continues carrying on The Bragg Healthy Lifestyle.

Paul C. Bragg and daughter Patricia express their opinions solely as Public Health Educators and Health Crusaders. They offer no cure for disease. Only the body has the ability to cure a person. Experts may disagree with some of the statements made in this book. However, such statements are considered to be factual, based on the long-time experience of dedicated pioneer Health Crusaders Paul C. Bragg and Patricia Bragg. If you suspect you have a medical problem, please always seek qualified Health Care professionals to help you make the healthiest, wisest and best-informed choices!

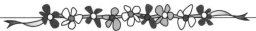

Count your blessings daily while you do your 30 to 45 minute brisk walks and exercises with these affirmations – health! strength! youth! vitality! peace! laughter! humility! understanding! forgiveness! joy! and love for eternity! and soon all these qualities will come flooding and bouncing into your life. With blessings of super health, peace and love to you, our dear friends – our readers. – Patricia Bragg, Health Crusader

If I were to name the three most precious resources of life, I would say books, friends and nature; and the greatest of these, at least the most constant and always at hand is Mother Nature and God. – John Burroughs

A Personal Message to Our Students
The Body Self-Cleans & Self-Heals When Given A Chance

It is our sincere desire that each one of our readers and students attain this precious super health and enjoy freedom from all nagging, tormenting human ailments. After studying this healthy Back and Foot Fitness Program, you can surmise that most physical problems arise from an unhealthy lifestyle that creates toxins throughout the body. Many of these trouble spots are years old and are often mainly concentrated in the intestines, colon and organs.

We have strived to teach you that there is no special diet for any one special ailment other than a diet rich in natural and organic live foods! The Bragg Healthy Lifestyle promotes cleansing through the eating of more organic raw fruits and vegetables combined with regular fasting. It is only through progressive cleansing that the human "cesspool" can be banished! During these cleansing times you might have weakness and might become discouraged! You may even go through healing crises from time to time. This is the time you must have great strength and faith! It is during these crises, when you feel the worst, that you are doing the greatest amount of deep detox cleansing. We promise you, it will be worth it!

You can create your own Garden of Eden anywhere you live, regardless of climate! All you have to do is to purify the body of its toxic poisons by living a healthy lifestyle! You can reach a stage of health and youthfulness that you never thought was possible! You can feel ageless where your chronological age actually stands still and pathological age will make you younger! When your body is free of deadly toxic material you will reach the physical, mental, emotional and spiritual state that will give you happiness every waking hour as it adds many more youthful, active, joyous years to your life!

With Blessings of Health, Peace & Love,

Patricia and Paul

236

BRAGG PHOTO GALLERY

PATRICIA & PAUL C. BRAGG, N.D., Ph.D.
Dynamic Daughter & Father are World Health Crusaders

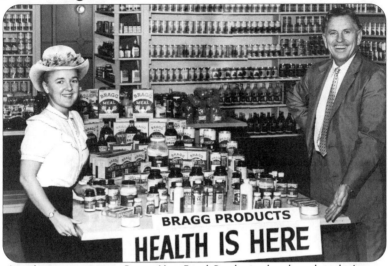

BRAGG PRODUCTS
HEALTH IS HERE

During the past century, Bragg Live Food Products developed and pioneered the very first line of Health Foods, from vitamins and minerals to organic nuts, seeds, and sun-dried fruits. This included over 365 health products, – *"one for each day of the year!"* says daughter Patricia Bragg.

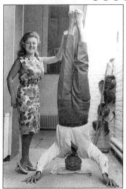

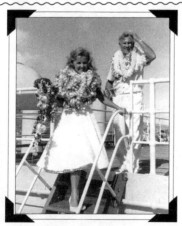

"Thanks for The Bragg Healthy Lifestyle that you shared with me and you are sharing with millions of others worldwide."
– John Gray, Ph.D., author

Picture from
People Magazine August, 1975.

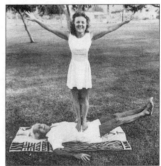

Patricia and father, Paul on world trip in 1950's, during stop in Tahiti.

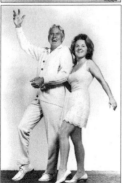

"You have recharged me with joy, hope, love and encouragement, which poured from your words. I am now fasting and using ACV. You have certainly improved my life!" – Marie Furia, New Jersey

Patricia Bragg stands on her father's stomach. Paul's stomach muscles are so strong he can lift Patricia up and down!

237

PHOTO GALLERY

PAUL C. BRAGG, N.D., Ph.D.
HEALTH CRUSADER
Life Extension Specialist and Originator of Health Food Stores

I have experienced a beautiful, remarkable, spiritual and physical awakening since reading Bragg Health Books. I'll never be the same again.
– Sandy Tuttle, Ohio

With every new day comes new strength and new thoughts.
– Eleanor Roosevelt

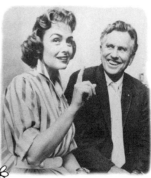

Actress Donna Reed saying "Health First" with Paul C. Bragg.

Dr. Paul C. Bragg (right) Creator Health Food Stores, Pioneer Life Extension Specialist, with his prize student Jack LaLanne. Paul started him on the royal road to health over 85 years ago!

Paul C. Bragg spent much of his time at the Hollywood Studios meeting with top Stars and motion picture industry executives, giving health lectures and private consultations. Dr. Paul C. Bragg was Hollywood's first highly respected, health, fitness and nutrition advisor to the Stars.

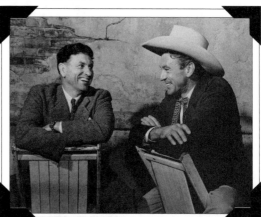

Paul C. Bragg with Gary Cooper, famous American film actor, best known for his many Western films.

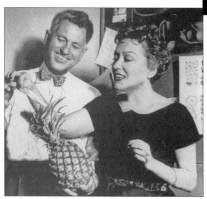

Paul C. Bragg with the famous Hollywood Actress Gloria Swanson, who was leading star in 20s, 30s and 40s. Gloria became a Bragg Health Devotee at 18 and she often would Health Crusade with Bragg during the 1950s.

238

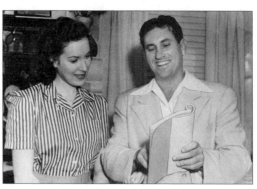

Maureen O'Hara and Paul C. Bragg. This Irish film actress and singer was best noted for playing in "Miracle on 34th Street" and "The Quiet Man."

PAUL C. BRAGG, N.D., Ph.D.
STAYING HEALTHY & FIT

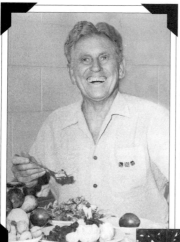

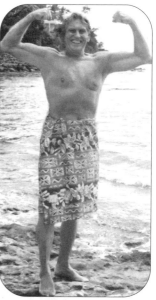

I'd like to thank you for teaching me how to take control of my health! I lost 55 pounds and I feel "great!" Bragg books have showed me vitality, happiness and being close to Mother Nature. You both are real "Crusaders for Health for the World."
Thanks!
– Leonard Amato

Dr. Paul C. Bragg and daughter Patricia were my early guiding inspiration to my health career.
– Jeffery Bland, Ph.D., Famous Food Scientist

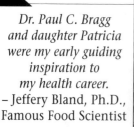

The best thing about the future is that it only comes one day at a time.
– Abraham Lincoln

Paul C. Bragg in Tahiti 1920's gathering tropical papaya fruit.

Paul C. Bragg owes his powerful body and superb health to living exclusively on live, vital, healthy, organic rich foods.

Dear Friends – you cannot know how greatly you have impacted my life and some of my friends! We love your Bragg Health Books, teachings and products and are now living healthier, happier lives. Thanks!
– Winnie Brown, Arizona

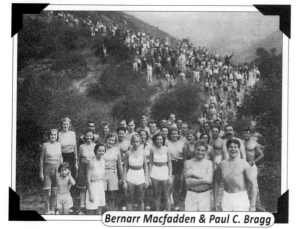

Bernarr Macfadden & Paul C. Bragg

A thousand happy Bragg Health Students enjoy hiking, exercise and fresh air on the trail to Mount Hollywood (above Griffith Observatory) in beautiful California, summer of 1932.

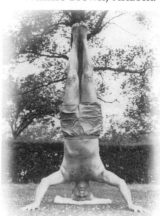

Paul C. Bragg exercising Regent's Park, London.

239

PAUL & PATRICIA BRAGG

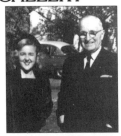

Patricia with 33rd President Harry S. Truman at his home in Independence, Missouri.

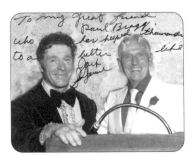

Paul C. Bragg, Creator of Health Food Stores, with his prize student Jack LaLanne, who thanks Bragg for saving his life at 15.

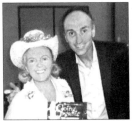

Patrica Bragg with Dr. Jeffrey Smith. He is leader in getting GMO's out of US foods. See GMO video by Jeffrey Smith and narrated by Lisa Oz (Dr. Oz's wife) on web: GeneticRouletteMovie.com

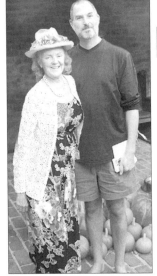

Patricia visiting with Steve Jobs at his home in Palo Alto during the Thanksgiving Holidays.

"I've been reading Bragg Books since high school. I'm thankful for the Bragg Healthy Lifestyle and admire their Health Crusading for a healthier, happier world."
– Steve Jobs, Creator –
Apple Computer

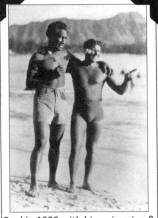

Paul in 1920 with his swimming & surfing friend, Duke Kahanamoku, Waikiki Beach, Diamond Head.

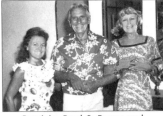

Patricia, Paul C. Bragg and Mrs. Duke (Nadine) Kahanamoku. (Nadine is Patricia's Godmother).

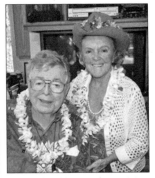

Dr. Earl Bakken with Patricia. He's famous for inventing the first Transistor Pacemaker. His firm Medtronic, developed it and a Resuscitator for fixing ailing hearts that have and are saving thousands of lives. Dr. Bakken lived in Hawaii.

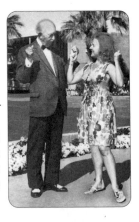

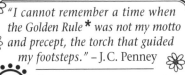

*"I cannot remember a time when the Golden Rule * was not my motto and precept, the torch that guided my footsteps."* – J.C. Penney

(240) *The Golden Rule: Do unto others as you would have them do unto you.

J.C. Penney & Patricia → exercising. They walked often in Palm Springs when he and his wife visited in the winter to enjoy the warm desert sunshine.

HEALTH CRUSADING TO HOLLYWOOD STARS

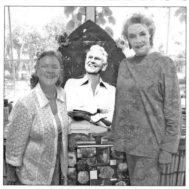

Patricia with friend Actress Jane Russell. Famous Hollywood Star of 40s to 60s.

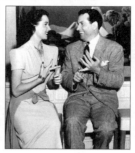

Jane Wyatt learning about health with Paul C. Bragg.

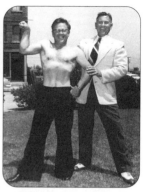

Mickey Rooney with Paul. Rooney was an American film actor and entertainer. He won multiple awards and had one of the longest careers of any actor to age 93!

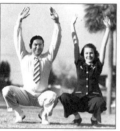

Paul C. Bragg exercising with Actress Helen Parrish.

"Thank you Paul & Patricia Bragg for my simple, easy-to-follow Healthy Lifestyle. You make my days healthy!" – Clint Eastwood, Academy Award Winning Film Producer, Director, Actor and Bragg follower for over 65 years.

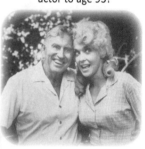

Paul C. Bragg and Donna Douglas, one of Hollywood's most beautiful and talented health advocates. She played the part of "Elly-May" in the Beverly Hillbillies, which became one of the longest-running series in television history and was the #1 show in America in its first 2 years.

Life is a Miracle Minute by Minute Year by Year!

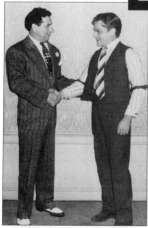

Paul C. Bragg with James Cagney, American film actor. He won major awards for wide variety of roles. The American Film Institute ranked Cagney 8th among the Greatest Male Hollywood Stars of All Time.

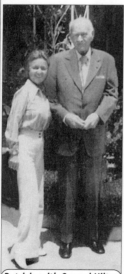

Patricia with Conrad Hilton

 Hotel founder, Conrad Hilton with Patricia Bragg, his Healthy Lifestyle Teacher. *"I wouldn't be alive today if it wasn't for the Braggs and their Bragg Healthy Lifestyle!"* – Conrad Hilton

"Thank you for your website. What a wealth of info to learn about how to live and eat healthy. Many Blessings!" – Michel & Mary, California

PAUL C. BRAGG, N.D., Ph.D.
PROMOTES HEALTH & FITNESS!

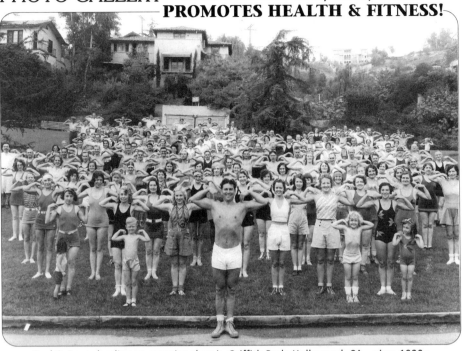

Paul C. Bragg leading an exercise class in Griffith Park, Hollywood, CA – circa 1920s.

Bragg Healthy Lifestyle works Miracles! – Jack LaLanne

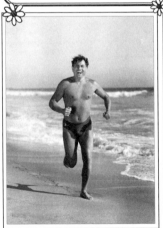

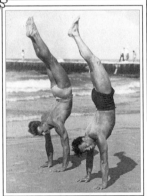

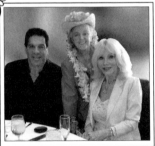

Patricia with Lou and wife Carla at Elaine LaLanne's 90th Birthday Party.

Friend and Paul C. Bragg doing handstand at the beach.

Paul running on Coney Island, New York, where he was a member of the Coney Island Polar Bear Club, known for Cold Water Swimming, 1930s.

TV Hulk Actor Lou Ferrigno gives thanks to Bragg Books. Lou went from puny to become Super Hulk! ➡

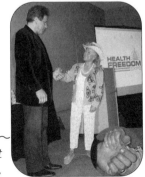

"I lost 102 lbs. with The Bragg Healthy Lifestyle and I have kept it off for over 15 years, staying away from white flour, sugar and other processed foods."– Dee McCaffrey, Chemist & Diet Counselor, Tempe, AZ

Lou & Patricia in Chicago Health Freedom Expo.

PATRICIA CONTINUING BRAGG HEALTH CRUSADE!

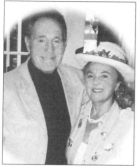

Jack LaLanne with Patricia.

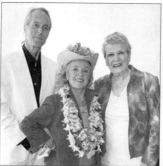

Jon & Elaine LaLanne with Patricia.

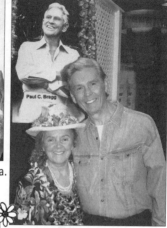

Mother Nature Loves US!

Patricia Bragg with Bill Galt inspired by Bragg Books, he founded Good Earth Restaurants.

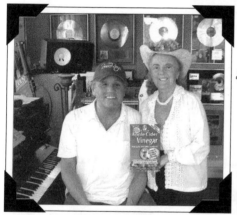

Patricia in studio with famous Beach Boy Bruce Johnston, Bragg follower over 40 years. He played for her their latest records.

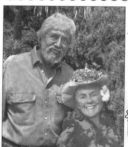

Patricia with Jean-Michel Cousteau Ocean Explorer & Environmentalist. OceanFutures.org

Enjoy a Lifetime of Radiant Health

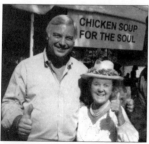

Patricia with Jack Canfield, Bragg follower, Motivational Speaker and Co-Producer of Chicken Soup For The Soul.

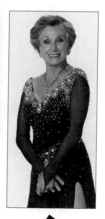

Patricia with Astronaut Buzz Aldrin, celebrating over 50 years since pilot of Apollo 11 first landed on the moon.

Famous Hollywood Actress Cloris Leachman, ardent health follower who sparkled with health and vitality said, *"The Miracle of Fasting Book is a miracle . . . it cured my asthma, my years of arthritis and many other health problems. I praise Paul and Patricia daily for their Health Crusading!"*

243

PHOTO GALLERY

PAUL & PATRICIA BRAGG HEALTH CRUSADING

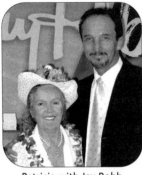

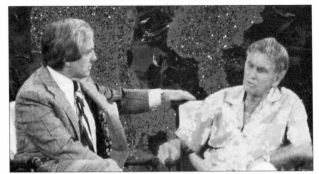

Patricia with Jay Robb.

Paul C. Bragg on the Merv Griffin Show, 1976.

Paul Bragg inspired me many years ago with The Miracle of Fasting Book and his pioneering philosophy on health. His daughter Patricia is a testament to the ageless value of living The Bragg Healthy Lifestyle. – Jay Robb, author of The Fruit Flush

During the many years Patricia worked with her father, she was right beside him, assisting him on Bragg Health Crusades worldwide. They were a great team, when you looked at them, you would see only two people headed in the same healthy direction!

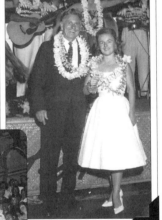

I am a big fan of Paul Bragg. I fast and follow The Bragg Healthy Lifestyle daily. The world and I are blessed with the health teachings of Paul and Patricia Bragg!
– Tony Robbins • TonyRobbins.com

✿ **Dream big, think big and enjoy the many miracles.** ✿

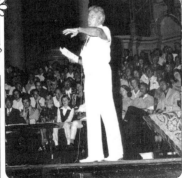

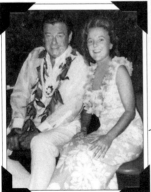

Paul & Daughter Patricia, Royal Hawaiian, Honolulu.

Paul – London Bragg Health Crusade.

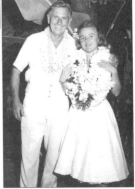

Actor Arthur Godfrey with Patricia, in Honolulu celebrating his 79th birthday.

Health Crusaders Paul C. Bragg and daughter Patricia traveled the world spreading health, inspiring millions to renew and revitalize their health.
Bragg Mottos:
3 John 2 and Genesis 6:3

(244)

100 YEAR HISTORY OF BRAGG HEALTH BOOKS & PRODUCTS

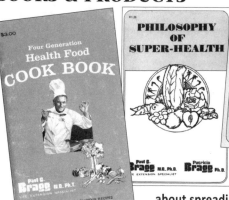

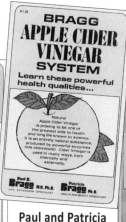

Paul and Patricia are passionate about spreading the message of health to the world.

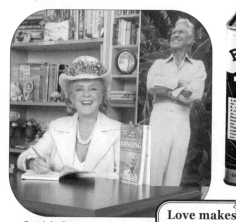

Patricia Bragg carries on her father's Health Legacy that he started over 100 years ago.

Love makes the World go 'round.

BRAGG TAVA
A delicious chocolate-flavored beverage. Contains vitamins A, B, C, B2, B6 and Iron.

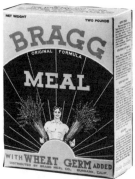

BRAGG MEAL CEREAL
Bragg was first to put wheat germ and 7 grains together for a delicious hot cereal.

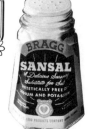

BRAGG SANSAL
A great Salt Substitute. This product was approved by Los Angeles Heart Assoc.

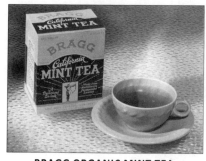

BRAGG ORGANIC MINT TEA
First Organic Herb Teas in America.

BRAGG 'E' WHEAT GERM OIL
Wheat germ oil with high Vitamin 'E' potency. Includes Omega-3 and Omega-6.

"Our lives have completely turned around! Our family is feeling so healthy, we must tell you about it." – Gene & Joan Zollner, parents of 11, Washington

245

HALL of LEGENDS
Patricia Bragg

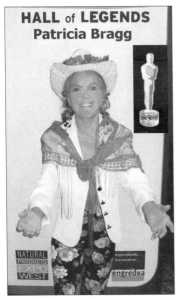

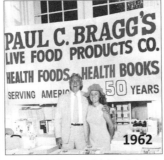

1962

Paul C. Bragg with Patricia, celebrating over 50 years of Bragg Health Products, Books & Crusading worldwide, spreading Health around the world.

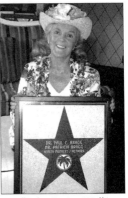

"Palm Spring Walk of Stars" – Patricia with Bragg Star.

Natural Foods Expo in Anaheim with 65,000 attendees from around the world honored Patricia Bragg and her father Paul C. Bragg as treasured Health Food Industry Legends.

BRAGG's 100th Anniversary Celebration

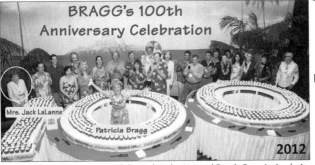

Mrs. Jack LaLanne

Patricia Bragg

2012

100 Year Anniversary Party celebrated at the Natural Foods Expo in Anaheim

Patricia, Staff & 1,000 Friends celebrated our 100 years of Bragg Healthy Products, Books & Health Crusading! We are proud Pioneers in this Big Health Industry that is helping to keep the world healthier! With Blessings of Health, Peace & Love to You!

Patricia

Bragg Hawaii Exercise Class was founded by Worldwide Health Crusader and Fitness Legend, Dr. Paul C. Bragg. He wanted to create a dynamic, Free Community Exercise Class, and he often taught these classes himself for many years. Patricia Bragg continues her father's health legacy by supporting the Bragg Exercise Class and participates in the class whenever she is in Hawaii.

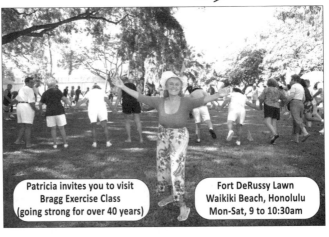

Patricia invites you to visit Bragg Exercise Class (going strong for over 40 years)

Fort DeRussy Lawn Waikiki Beach, Honolulu Mon-Sat, 9 to 10:30am

"Please make a record of your family history & background. Take pictures – make your own 'Photo Gallery'. Take videos – make movies of your children, spouse, mother and father, family gatherings, etc. These memories are precious & important to save for future generations." – Patricia Bragg

BRAGG BACK & FOOT
Fitness Program

Index

Index

Dream big, think big, but enjoy the small miracles of everyday life!

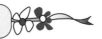

What sunshine is to flowers, smiles are to humanity. – Joseph Addison

Index

Prayer is the mortar that holds our house together. – Mother Teresa

Apple Cider Vinegar - Miracle Health System

BY PAUL C. BRAGG, N.D., PH.D.
and PATRICIA BRAGG

Paul C. Bragg, originator of health stores in America, and world-renowned health crusader Patricia Bragg, introduced America to the life-changing value of Apple Cider Vinegar, with the miracle enzyme known as "the mother." Now a widely popular beverage, this book reveals the legendary health-and life-giving versatility of apple cider vinegar. Following in the footsteps of Hippocrates, who taught the benefits of ACV to his patients in 400 BC, the Braggs teach dozens of reasons to use vinegar, including as a beauty aid, for skin treatments, in recipes, as an antibiotic, anti-septic, hair-revitalizing rinse, headache reliever, and weight reducer. ACV optimizes digestive health and can reduce or eliminate acid reflux. Paul and Patricia Bragg have helped millions heal and restore their vitality and zest for life through their time-tested understanding of natural health. *Apple Cider Vinegar: Miracle Health System* is informative, entertaining, and invaluable for anyone wanting to feel their best.

Bragg Healthy Lifestyle - Vital Living at Any Age

BY PAUL C. BRAGG, N.D., PH.D.
and PATRICIA BRAGG

Learn the simple strategies of radical health and vibrant wellness that The Bragg Healthy Lifestyle has brought to millions! What is an ageless body? For health pioneers Paul C. Bragg and Patricia Bragg, an ageless body sparkles with vitality, immune strength, mental clarity, and digestive ease. The Braggs teach why a toxic-free diet maximizes energy, supports weight loss, and can help heal illness and disease. In the newly revised *Bragg Healthy Lifestyle: Vital Living At Any Age*, the trailblazing father-daughter team who alerted us nearly a century ago to the dangers of sugar and toxic foods, detail every key aspect of creating and maintaining ageless health, including detoxification, stress-release, nutrition, exercise and the importance of taking charge of not only what goes into our bodies, but practices such as fasting, which release the toxins that may unnecessarily accelerate the aging process. "You are what you eat, drink, breathe, think, say and do," is the Bragg motto. From the foods we eat to our outlook, the environments we live in and even in our physical activities, the authors encourage readers to replace toxins with nutrients, flush out poisons and waste efficiently, exercise, breathe deeply and well, and cultivate happiness and harmony in our daily lives.

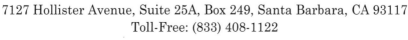

Bragg Books are available at most Health & Book Stores – Nationwide

HEALTH SCIENCE
7127 Hollister Avenue, Suite 25A, Box 249, Santa Barbara, CA 93117
Toll-Free: (833) 408-1122

The Miracle of Fasting - Proven Throughout History

BY PAUL C. BRAGG, N.D., PH.D.
and PATRICIA BRAGG

In this newly revised best-seller, known to millions as the "bible of fasting" health pioneers and researchers Paul C. Bragg and Patricia Bragg teach why this ancient practice is key to health and energy, and critical to longevity and ageless vitality, due to our toxic environment and the stress of our daily lives. They share a detailed, step-by-step approach, accessible and informative for both beginners and experienced fasters. Our bodies must process not only our food and water, but the air we breathe, and whatever chemicals they may contain. Since detoxification and digestion take more energy than even strenuous athletic pursuits, fasting allows the mind and body to rest, renew and regenerate, to come into harmony and balance, and release the effects of stimulating foods like caffeine and sugars. The goal of fasting, say the authors, is to allow for the mind and body to self-heal. This concise, tightly edited *The Miracle of Fasting* is filled with personal stories of Paul C. Bragg's travels around the world, including a fasting journey in India with Mahatma Gandhi.

Healthy Heart - Learn the Facts

BY PAUL C. BRAGG, N.D., PH.D.
and PATRICIA BRAGG

Heart disease claims more American lives than any other illness and is the number one cause of death for women. World-renowned health pioneers Paul C. Bragg and Patricia Bragg teach time-tested, proven strategies for healing and maintaining a healthy heart for a long, active life! In a world filled with technological wizardry and products, the human heart still outperforms them all. That is – if that human heart is kept healthy. That is what the trailblazers Paul C. Bragg and Patricia Bragg have done in this book, sharing simple suggestions for lifestyle changes, nutritional support and exercises that will keep this most miraculous machine, your body, healthy and strong. You will learn how the heart works and how and why coronary disease is preventable and reversible. The authors provide an easy-to-follow blueprint for heart health that includes stress-release techniques, affirming that a positive mental outlook on life is a major element of heart health. The Braggs are legendary in the field of nutrition and health, and this newly revised and edited edition is a foundation of The Bragg Healthy Lifestyle. It is one of the most comprehensive heart health books on the market today.

HEALTH SCIENCE
7127 Hollister Avenue, Suite 25A, Box 249, Santa Barbara, CA 93117
Toll-Free: (833) 408-1122

Building Powerful Nerve Force & Positive Energy - Reduce Stress, Worry and Anger

BY PAUL C. BRAGG, N.D., PH.D.
and PATRICIA BRAGG

What is Nerve Force and why should you care about it? According to mental health trailblazers Paul C. Bragg and Patricia Bragg, "Nerve Force" is a type of life energy stored in the nerves, muscles, organs, and brain. The more Nerve Force you have, the quicker you can re-charge it, and the healthier, happier, and more satisfying a life you will lead. If you suffer from burnout, stress, fatigue, anxiety, insomnia or depression, this book is for you! We know that the ability to feel joy and peace is essential to a complete experience of vitality and wellness. Our thoughts, our attitudes, our outlook, and our emotional well-being are all dependent on having a powerful "Nerve Force." Just like any muscle that we can develop and strengthen, we can build our Nerve Force so that we are resilient, relaxed, and calm, even during times of stress. Paul C. Bragg and Patricia Bragg show you how with simple mental exercises and suggestions for specific foods that replenish your Nerve Force, as well as foods that deplete it, in this newly revised edition of *Building Powerful Nerve Force & Positive Energy* the father-daughter team explains to readers the reward of paying attention to the energy that is responsible for not only our physical capabilities and our vital body functions, but our ability to process information and feel centered and grounded, no matter what life throws at us. They teach us that maintaining a healthy Nerve Force, leads to a balanced and fruitful life.

Super Power Breathing - For Optimum Health & Healing

BY PAUL C. BRAGG, N.D., PH.D.
and PATRICIA BRAGG

Do you sometimes find that you are panting instead of breathing? Many of us do! This can cause headaches, anxiety, fatigue, and brain fog. The quality of our breath determines the quality of our life! This book teaches us how to breathe in a way that replenishes the body with the oxygen it so deeply craves. "The more effectively we breathe, the more effectively we live," write the authors, world-renowned health pioneers Paul C. Bragg and Patricia Bragg. "Super Power Breathing can make your life-force stronger, calmer and smarter." The Super Power Breathing program has been followed by Olympic athletes and millions of Bragg followers, and is filled with simple exercises for energizing and rejuvenating your breath, and your whole body. Research shows that we use only one-fourth to one-half of our lung capacity with each breath. This starves our body much like if we are depriving it of food. We are slowly robbing our body of its most vital, invisible nourishment – oxygen. In its newly revised form, the Bragg Super Power Breathing Program will give you all the tools you need to shift from shallow breathing to taking deep, oxygen-filled, life-giving breaths!

Authored by America's First Family of Health
Live Longer – Healthier – Stronger Self-Improvement Library

Water - The Shocking Truth

BY PAUL C. BRAGG, N.D., PH.D.
and PATRICIA BRAGG

The water you drink can literally make or break your health. The purity of our water is the most critical element in maintaining radical vitality, and healing from illness and disease. In this newly revised edition of *Water: The Shocking Truth*, health crusaders Paul C. Bragg and Patricia Bragg reveal the dangers of tap water, which research shows can be responsible for many ailments, due to the addition of dangerous chemicals such as fluoride and chlorine. In this book, the trailblazing father-daughter team teach the many functions water performs in the body, from regulating the various systems to flushing the body of waste and toxins. But what if the substance we use to cleanse our bodies is itself polluted? With the mandatory fluoridation of water in the municipal water systems, the authors assert that has been the case for decades. Added to the public water supply to prevent tooth decay starting in the 1950s, fluoride has long been known to be a toxin, used in pesticides and rat poisons. Learn what types of water are optimal to drink, how and why to detox your body with nature's most life-giving liquid, and the health-and-life-saving value of installing a water filter in your shower!

Bragg Back & Foot Fitness Program - Keys to a Pain-Free Back & Strong Healthy Feet

BY PAUL C. BRAGG, N.D., PH.D.
and PATRICIA BRAGG

If you are suffering with back or foot pain, look no further for a comprehensive program that will restore health to the parts of your body that carry you through life! Remember when we were children, and we had the kind of energy and flexibility to play for hours? Agile and active, we could twist, bend, stretch and climb with little effort. However, hours looking at a computer screen, a sedentary lifestyle and poor posture can take their toll. Eventually our backs start to hurt and cramp with every movement, and our feet ache after just a short walk. We start feeling "old." In *Bragg Back & Foot Fitness Program*, the father-daughter team of world-renowned health pioneers, Paul C. Bragg and Patricia Bragg teach how to speed the healing of injuries and develop a strong and flexible back and healthy feet, rejuvenating and re-energizing our bodies in the process. The trailblazing health experts who brought wellness and vitality to millions, including fitness guru Jack LaLanne, outline the keys to a healthy spine, pain-free back and bunion-free feet through nutritional support and clearly illustrated, simple exercises, as well as other tips for posture and massage. Paul and Patricia Bragg reveal the healing properties of herbs, effective ways to practice foot reflexology, how to deal with arthritis, athlete's foot, plantar fasciitis, and foot problems caused by diabetes. By following the authors' Back and Foot Care Program, you (256) can begin to treat your body as Mother Nature intended you to, and creating painless feet, a strong back and a powerful body will begin!

PATRICIA BRAGG
Health Crusader and "Angel of Health and Healing"

Author, Lecturer, Nutritionist, Health & Lifestyle Educator to World Leaders, Hollywood Stars, Singers, Athletes & Millions.

Patricia is a life-long health advocate and activist, admired internationally for her passionate work promoting healthy living. For many years she traveled the world, teaching The Bragg Healthy Lifestyle for physical, spiritual, emotional health and joy. She was invited to give lectures, visited radio shows, was profiled in magazines and appealed to people of all ages, nationalities and walks-of-life. Together with Paul, she co-authored a collection of ten books, with inspiration and techniques for living a long, vital, happy life. Now in her 90s and living on an organic farm in California, Patricia herself is a testament to these teachings and the sparkling symbol of health, perpetual youth and radiant energy.

PAUL C. BRAGG, N.D., Ph.D.
Life Extension Specialist • World Health Crusader
Lecturer and Advisor to Olympic Athletes, Royalty, Stars & Millions.
Originator of Health Food Stores & Founder of Health Movement Worldwide

---

Paul C. Bragg was at the forefront of the modern health movement, having inspired generations to turn toward wellness. At a young age, Paul turned his own health around by developing an eating, breathing and exercise program to build strength and vitality. From this life-changing experience, he pledged to dedicate the rest of his life to promoting a healthy lifestyle. He opened one of the country's first health food stores, which eventually led to the creation of the Bragg Live Foods company. With a devoted following, Paul traveled giving lectures and sharing his expertise, while serving as an advisor to athletes and movie stars alike. Even Jack LaLanne, the original television fitness guru, credited Paul with having introduced him to the importance of healthy living. In addition to the books Paul wrote with Patricia, they co-hosted television and radio shows and worked together to bring wellness to the world. Paul himself excelled in athletics, loved the ocean and the outdoors, and radiated with health and a warm smile.

Patricia inspires you to Renew, Rejuvenate and Revitalize your Life with "The Bragg Healthy Lifestyle" Books. Millions have benefitted from these life-changing philosophies with a longer, healthier, happier life!

Take Time for 12 Things

1. Take time to **Work** –
   it is the price of success.
2. Take time to **Think** –
   it is the source of power.
3. Take time to **Play** –
   it is the secret of youth.
4. Take time to **Read** –
   it is the foundation of knowledge.
5. Take time to **Worship** –
   it is the highway of reverence and
   washes the dust of earth from our eyes.
6. Take time to **Help and Enjoy Friends** –
   it is the source of happiness.
7. Take time to **Love and Share** –
   it is the one sacrament of life.
8. Take time to **Dream** –
   it hitches the soul to the stars.
9. Take time to **Laugh** –
   it is the singing that helps life's loads.
10. Take time for **Beauty** –
    it is everywhere in nature.
11. Take time for **Health** –
    it is the true wealth and treasure of life.
12. Take time to **Plan** –
    it is the secret of being able to have time
    for the first 11 things.

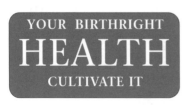

YOUR BIRTHRIGHT
HEALTH
CULTIVATE IT

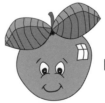

Have an
Apple
Healthy Life!

3 John 2

Teach me thy way, LORD, lead me in a straight path,
because of my oppressors. – Psalm 27:11